Reason to Change

Rational Emotive Behaviour Therapy (REBT) is an approach to counselling and psychotherapy in which great emphasis is placed on how emotional problems are determined by thoughts, beliefs and behaviour. However, no book before has taught the skills needed to use this therapeutic approach in practice in a thorough and accessible way.

Reason to Change is the first major workbook which teaches the practical skills of REBT. Each skill is explained in detail, and examples are given of how each skill can be put into practice. These skills include:

- developing a problem list and setting goals
- choosing a target problem and assessing a specific example
- questioning beliefs
- dealing with doubts, reservations and objections
- taking action.

By using these skills in an active way, it can be possible to overcome emotional problems such as anxiety, depression, shame, guilt, hurt, unhealthy anger, unhealthy jealousy and unhealthy envy. This book can be used by people on their own, and by those who are consulting an REBT therapist. It will also be of interest to therapists and counsellors.

Windy Dryden is an REBT therapist and Professor of Counselling at Goldsmiths College, University of London. He has written or edited numerous books, including *Four Approaches to Counselling and Psychotherapy, On Becoming a Psychotherapist* and *Adult Clinical Problems*.

Reason to Change

■ A Rational Emotive Behaviour Therapy (REBT) Workbook

Windy Dryden

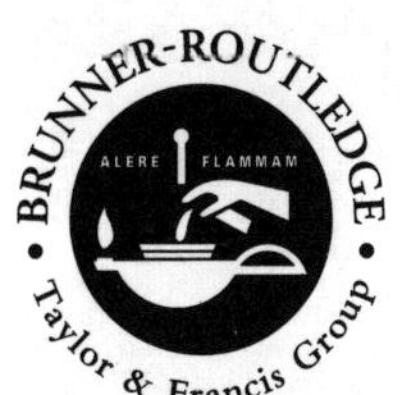

First published 2001 by Brunner-Routledge
27 Church Road, Hove, East Sussex BN3 2FA

Simultaneously published in the USA and Canada
by Taylor & Francis Inc
325 Chestnut Street, Philadelphia PA 19106

Brunner-Routledge is an imprint of the Taylor & Francis Group

Typeset in Century Old Style by Keystroke,
Jacaranda Lodge, Wolverhampton
Printed and bound in Great Britain by
TJ International, Padstow, Cornwall
Cover design by Terry Foley

British Library Cataloguing in Publication Data
A catalogue record for this book is available from the British Library

Library of Congress Cataloging-in-Publication Data
Dryden, Windy.
Reason to change : a rational emotive behaviour therapy (REBT) workbook / Windy Dryden.
p. cm.
Includes bibliographical references and index.
1. Rational-emotive psychotherapy. I. Title: Rational emotive behaviour therapy (REBT) workbook. II. Title.

RC489.R3 D793 2001
616.89′14–dc21 2001025531

ISBN 0–415–22980–4

Contents

Figures and tables

Figures

Tables

Preface

Rational Emotive Behaviour Therapy (REBT) is an approach to counselling and psychotherapy that falls fairly and squarely within the cognitive-behavioural therapeutic tradition (CBT) that is currently in vogue. In this tradition great emphasis is placed on the role that thoughts, beliefs and behaviour play in the development and maintenance of emotional problems.

It is generally recognized that REBT was the first CBT approach to make an impact on the world's therapeutic stage. Its founder, Albert Ellis who originated REBT in 1955, is regarded as one of the two grandfathers of the CBT movement (Aaron Beck, the founder of cognitive therapy, being the other). You may like to know that I have trained with both Ellis and Beck but see myself very much as an REBT therapist.

Indeed, I have been practising REBT since 1977 and have written many books on the subject. This book, however, is very different from my other REBT books in that here I have attempted to teach, in a very specific way, the skills that you need to acquire if you are to get the most from this therapeutic approach.

While I have written this workbook so that it can be used by people on their own, it can also be used by those who are consulting an REBT therapist. To get the most from the book, though, it is important that you don't just read it. Rather, use the skills in an active way to help yourself overcome your emotional problems. To help you do this I have explained each skill in detail and have provided an example of how each skill has been put into practice. Feel free to photocopy the forms as you work through the book.

I have written this book primarily for people whose emotional problems *interfere* with the quality of their lives. If this fits your situation you can use this book on your own or while consulting an REBT therapist. However, if your problems *disable* rather than just interfere with your life, do not use this workbook on your own. Consult an REBT therapist and use it in conjunction with such consultations (see Appendix 3 to find out how to contact an REBT therapist in your area). If you are in doubt about this issue, talk it over in the first instance with your GP.

While this workbook has many advantages, it also has a distinct drawback. It has not been and could not have been written in a way that is tailor made to help you overcome your particular emotional problems. While I have tried to anticipate your questions and to answer them in a clear, straightforward way, it is likely that you may have questions about the material in this book that I have not dealt with. If you accept this limitation and go forward despite it then I am hopeful that you will derive much benefit from the exercises that I describe within these pages, particularly if you commit yourself to the process.

Lack of space prevents me from giving you detailed suggestions to help you deal with each of the eight disturbed emotions for which people seek therapeutic help: anxiety, depression, shame, guilt, hurt, unhealthy anger, unhealthy jealousy and unhealthy envy. However, in Appendix 4, I provide reading suggestions for most of these problematic emotions. You can use this workbook in conjunction with such reading since the texts dovetail very well.

You may be wondering why I have called this workbook *Reason to Change*. The answer is twofold, first, in order to change you need to have a reason to change, and second, you need to use your reason to change!

I hope that you benefit from using this workbook and as I say at the end, I would be very interested to learn of your experiences in doing so. Good luck!

Windy Dryden

Chapter 1

The REBT view of psychological problems

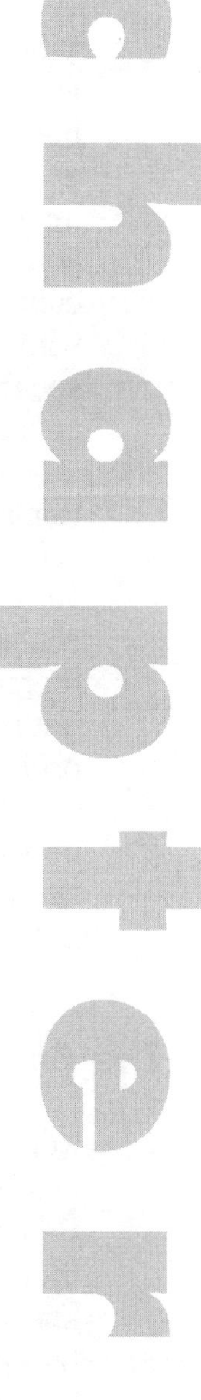

The importance of informed consent

When you consult a professionally trained counsellor or psychotherapist, it is likely that he or she will belong to a recognized professional body and that body will have a code of ethics and practice that your counsellor is expected to abide by. One of the principles in this code is known as the principle of informed consent. This principle states that it is a mark of ethical practice that you should give your informed consent to a therapeutic approach before your counsellor or psychotherapist proceeds to help you by using this approach with you. If we look at the principle of informed consent carefully, we quickly see that in order for you to give your consent to proceed with an approach to counselling/psychotherapy you have to be informed about it.

When you consult a rational emotive behaviour therapist, one of the first things that he or she will do is to explain to you something about Rational Emotive Behaviour Therapy (henceforth called REBT) so that you can make an informed decision whether to proceed with this approach or whether to consult a therapist from a different therapeutic persuasion. Now, your REBT therapist is unlikely to overwhelm you with too much information about REBT. Rather, he or she will tell you something about the REBT view of psychological problems and something about how the approach is practised.

Let me relate an incident from my own practice that underscores the importance of the counsellor explaining something about the approach that he or she practises as a prelude to gaining the person's informed consent to proceed with the approach or not.

The Birmingham episode

Many years ago (in the late 1970s) when I lived and worked in Birmingham, a man rang to ask whether I practised 'RT'. Now, REBT (Rational Emotive Behaviour Therapy) used to be called RT (Rational Therapy) until 1961, so I thought that this man had read some old material written when REBT was known as RT. Anyway, when he came to his first appointment I explained to him the REBT view of psychological problems even though I thought (as it turned out wrongly) that he had already made an informed decision to seek me out because I practised REBT/RT.

After I had explained to him the REBT view of psychological problems (which I will outline for you in the next section), he looked puzzled and exclaimed that he had never heard such intellectualized clap-trap. It transpired that he was looking for a practitioner of a very different kind of RT, known as Reichian Therapy, a therapeutic approach based on the release of energy blockages in the body by deep massage and other physical procedures. So without more ado I referred him to a local Reichian Therapist whom, as I later discovered, he found very helpful.

This is why it is important for me to spell out for you the REBT view of psychological problems even if you think you understand what this view is. This is how *I* know that the consent you will give to proceed with this workbook is informed.

As I mentioned in the preface to this text, you may be using this workbook either in conjunction with consultations with an REBT therapist or on your own as a self-help manual. Either way, in this chapter, I am going to explain the REBT view of psychological problems and, in the next chapter, I will discuss some of the fundamentals of REBT practice so that you have sufficient information about REBT either to give your informed consent to proceed with this workbook or to seek a different kind of help if it transpires that REBT is not the approach to counselling or self-help that you are looking for.

There is a viewpoint in American social work that captures this point nicely. This viewpoint states that when you seek help, from a counsellor for example, you have the status of an 'applicant'. You become a 'client' when you give your informed consent to proceed with the counselling. Thus, at the moment, you are an applicant. I hope that after you have read what I have had to say about the REBT view of psychological problems (in this chapter) and how REBT addresses these problems (in the next chapter), you will become a client. If not, and you decide to seek a different approach to counselling, I wish you well and suggest that you consult a book that I wrote with a colleague of mine, Colin Feltham, entitled *Counselling and Psychotherapy: A Consumer's Guide* (Dryden and Feltham, 1995), which tells you something about different approaches to counselling and psychotherapy.

The 'Giving a Speech' model

Let me begin by inviting you to join me as a participant as I go over the 'Giving a Speech' model. This model gets to the heart of REBT's view of psychological problems. There are four steps to this model.

Step 1

I want you to imagine that you have been asked by your boss to give a speech to a group of visiting dignitaries (the first half of which will be before their morning coffee break and the second half after it) and you hold the following belief about this event:

> I want to give a good speech, but it isn't absolutely necessary for me to do so. If I don't give a good speech, it will be bad, but it wouldn't be the end of the world.

How would you feel about the possibility of not giving a good speech while holding this belief?

If you think about it you would probably feel concerned about the possibility of not giving a good speech, but you wouldn't feel unduly anxious about it.

Step 2

Now, in this second step, I want you to imagine again that you have been asked by your boss to give a speech to a group of visiting dignitaries (the first half of which will be before their morning coffee break and the second half after it), but this time you hold the following different belief about this event:

> I absolutely must give a good speech and it would be truly awful if I didn't.

How would you feel this time about the possibility of not giving a good speech while holding this different belief?

If you think about it you would probably feel very anxious about the possibility of not giving a good speech.

Now I want you to focus on one important point here:

> While facing the same event, your different feelings are determined by different beliefs.

Step 3

In the third step of the model I want you to imagine that you still believe that you absolutely have to give a good speech and it would be terrible if you didn't. You give the first half of your speech and at the end of it you conclude that it has gone down well. Now, how would you feel about that? You would probably feel relieved or pleased.

Step 4

But, still believing that you have to give a good speech and it would be awful if you didn't, you suddenly stop feeling relieved or pleased and become anxious again. What do you think you would be anxious about?

That's right, you would probably be anxious about the possibility that the second half of your speech wouldn't be good.

Conclusion

The point of this model is the following:

> That all humans, black or white, rich or poor, male or female, from whichever culture make themselves emotionally disturbed when they don't get what they demand they must get and are vulnerable to emotional disturbance when they do get what they demand because the situation may change and their demands may no longer be met. However, if humans stayed with their preferences and didn't change these into demands, then they would still experience negative feelings when their preferences weren't met, but these negative feelings would be healthy and would motivate them to change what can be changed and adjust constructively to what can't be changed.

Have you ever heard the famous dictum attributed to Epictetus, the Stoic philosopher: 'People are disturbed not by things, but by their views of things'? The REBT view of psychological problems is very nicely summarized by a re-formulation of this dictum, namely:

> People are disturbed, not by things, but by their rigid and extreme views of things.

Let me now consider more formally the rigid and extreme beliefs (henceforth referred to as irrational beliefs) that REBT holds are at the core of many psychological problems and the alternative flexible and non-extreme beliefs (henceforth referred to as rational beliefs) that are at the core of healthy psychological responses.

Irrational beliefs and their rational alternatives

Irrational beliefs are evaluative ideas that have the following characteristics, they are:

1 rigid or extreme;
2 inconsistent with reality;
3 illogical or nonsensical; and they
4 lead largely to dysfunctional consequences.

On the other hand, rational beliefs have the following characteristics, they are:

1 flexible or non-extreme;
2 consistent with reality;

3 logical or sensible; and they
4 lead largely to functional consequences.

REBT theory posits four irrational beliefs and their rational alternatives.

Demands versus full preferences

Demands

Demands are rigid ideas that people hold about how things absolutely must or must not be. Demands can be placed on:

- oneself, e.g. 'I must do well';
- others, e.g. 'You must treat me well';
- life conditions, e.g. 'Life must be fair'.

Ellis's view is that of all the irrational beliefs that I will discuss in this chapter, it is these demands that are at the very core of many psychological problems. The healthy alternative to a demand is a full preference.

Full preferences

Full preferences are flexible ideas that people hold about how they would like things to be without demanding that they have to be that way. Full preferences can relate to:

- oneself, e.g. 'I want to do well, but I don't have to do so';
- others, e.g. 'I want you to treat me well, but unfortunately you don't have to do so';
- life conditions, e.g. 'I very much want life to be fair, but unfortunately it doesn't have to be the way I want it to be'.

Again, Ellis's position is that of all the rational beliefs that I will discuss in this chapter, it is these full preferences that are at the very core of healthy psychological responses to negative life events.

Awfulizing beliefs versus anti-awfulizing beliefs

Awfulizing beliefs

Awfulizing beliefs are extreme ideas that people hold as derivatives from their demands when these demands aren't met. For example:

- 'I must do well *and it's terrible if I don't*';
- 'You must treat me well *and it's awful when you don't*';
- 'Life must be fair *and it's the end of the world when it's not*'.

An awfulizing belief stems from the demand that things must not be as bad as they are and is extreme in the sense that the person believes at the time one or more of the following:

1. nothing could be worse;
2. the event in question is worse than 100 per cent bad;
3. no good could possibly come from this bad event.

The healthy alternative to an awfulizing belief is an anti-awfulizing belief.

Anti-awfulizing beliefs

Anti-awfulizing beliefs are non-extreme ideas that people hold as derivatives from their full preferences when these full preferences aren't met. For example:

- 'I want to do well but I don't have to do so, *it's bad if I don't do well but not terrible*';
- 'I want you to treat me well but unfortunately you don't have to do so, *when you don't treat me well it's really unfortunate but not awful*';
- 'I very much want life to be fair but unfortunately it doesn't have to be the way I want it to be, *if life is unfair that's very bad, but not the end of the world*'.

An anti-awfulizing belief stems from the full preference that I'd like things not to be as bad as they are, but that doesn't mean that they must not be and it is non-extreme in the sense that the person believes at the time one or more of the following:

1. things could always be worse;
2. the event in question is less than 100 per cent bad;
3. good could come from this bad event.

Low frustration tolerance beliefs versus high frustration tolerance beliefs

Low frustration tolerance beliefs

Low frustration tolerance beliefs are extreme ideas that people hold as derivatives from their demands when these demands aren't met. For example:

- 'I must do well *and I can't bear it if I don't*';
- 'You must treat me well *and it's intolerable when you don't*';
- 'Life must be fair *and I can't stand it when it's not*'.

A low frustration tolerance stems from the demand that things must not be as frustrating or uncomfortable as they are and is extreme in the sense that the person believes at the time one or both of the following:

1 I will die or disintegrate if the frustration or discomfort continues to exist;
2 I will lose the capacity to experience happiness if the frustration or discomfort continues to exist.

The healthy alternative to a low frustration tolerance belief is a high frustration tolerance belief.

High frustration tolerance beliefs

High frustration tolerance beliefs are non-extreme ideas that people hold as derivatives from their full preferences when these full preferences aren't met. For example:

- 'I want to do well but I don't have to do so, *when I don't do well it is difficult to bear but I can bear it and it's worth bearing*';
- 'I want you to treat me well but unfortunately you don't have to do so, *when you don't treat me well it's really hard to tolerate but I can tolerate it and it's worth it to me to do so*';
- 'I very much want life to be fair but unfortunately it doesn't have to be the way I want it to be, *if life is unfair that's hard to stand but I can stand it and it is in my best interests to do so*'.

A high frustration tolerance belief stems from the full preference that it is undesirable when things are as frustrating or uncomfortable as they are, but unfortunately things don't have to be different. It is non-extreme in the sense that the person believes at the time one or more of the following:

1 I will struggle if the frustration or discomfort continues to exist, but I will neither die nor disintegrate;
2 I will not lose the capacity to experience happiness if the frustration or discomfort continues to exist, although this capacity will be temporarily diminished;
3 the frustration or discomfort is worth tolerating.

Depreciation beliefs versus acceptance beliefs

Depreciation beliefs

Depreciation beliefs are extreme ideas that people hold about self, other(s) and the world as derivatives from their demands when these demands aren't met. For example:

- 'I must do well *and I am a failure if I don't*';
- 'You must treat me well *and you are a bad person if you don't*';
- 'Life must be fair *and the world is bad if it isn't*'.

A depreciation belief stems from the demand that I, you or things must be as I want them to be and is extreme in the sense that the person believes at the time one or more of the following:

1 a person can legitimately be given a single global rating that defines their essence and one's worth is dependent upon conditions that change (e.g. my worth goes up when I do well and goes down when I don't do well);
2 the world can legitimately be given a single rating that defines its essential nature and the value of the world varies according to what happens within it (e.g. the value of the world goes up when something fair occurs and goes down when something unfair happens);
3 you can legitimately rate a person on the basis of his or her discrete aspects;
4 you can legitimately rate the world on the basis of its discrete aspects.

The healthy alternative to a depreciation belief is an acceptance belief.

Acceptance beliefs

Acceptance beliefs are non-extreme ideas that people hold as derivatives from their full preferences when these full preferences aren't met. For example:

- 'I want to do well but I don't have to do so, *when I don't do well I am not a failure, I am a fallible human being who is not doing well on this occasion*';
- 'I want you to treat me well but unfortunately you don't have to do so, *when you don't treat me well you are not a bad person, rather a fallible human being who is treating me poorly*';
- 'I very much want life to be fair but unfortunately it doesn't have to be the way I want it to be, *if life is unfair it is only unfair in this respect and doesn't prove that the world is a rotten place. The world is a complex place where many good, bad and neutral things happen*'.

An acceptance belief is non-extreme in the sense that the person believes at the time one or more of the following:

1 A person cannot legitimately be given a single global rating that defines their essence and one's worth, as far as one has it, is not dependent upon conditions that change (e.g. my worth stays the same whether or not I do well);
2 The world cannot legitimately be given a single rating that defines its essential nature and the value of the world does not vary according to what happens within it (e.g. the value of the world stays the same whether fairness exists at any given time or not);
3 It makes sense to rate discrete aspects of a person and of the world, but it does not make sense to rate a person or the world on the basis of these discrete aspects.

The effects of irrational beliefs and their rational alternatives

Holding irrational beliefs about life's adversities has a number of deleterious effects on your psychological functioning.

- Irrational beliefs lead you to have one of a number of unhealthy negative emotions such as anxiety, depression, guilt, shame, hurt, unhealthy anger, unhealthy jealousy and unhealthy envy about negative life events.
- Irrational beliefs lead you to act in a number of self-, other- and relationship-defeating ways.
- Irrational beliefs have an impairing impact on the way you subsequently think. Thus, they lead you to think unrealistically about yourself, others and the world. For example, irrational beliefs are often the breeding ground for what are called cognitive distortions. Thus, if you believe that you must perform well in public and you think that you haven't, then you are likely to think in a variety of distorted ways, for example mind-reading (e.g. 'I'm sure that the audience think that I made a fool of

myself), overgeneralization ('I'll always do poorly in public situations') and minimization ('there were no redeeming features to my presentation'). Irrational beliefs also have an effect on what you attend to and what you recall from your memory. Thus, when there is a possibility that a threat may occur to something of value in your personal domain and you hold an irrational belief about this threat, then your attention will be drawn to the existence of the threat and you may exaggerate (a) the chances that the threat will occur, and (b) the nature of the threat itself. Also, when you have experienced a significant loss to your personal domain and hold an irrational belief about this loss, then you will tend to remember other losses rather than the gains that you have experienced in your life.

By contrast, holding rational beliefs about the same adversities has a number of productive effects on your psychological functioning.

- Rational beliefs lead you to have one of a number of healthy negative emotions such as concern, sadness, remorse, disappointment, sorrow, healthy anger, healthy jealousy and healthy envy about negative life events.
- Rational beliefs lead you to act in a number of self-, other- and relationship-enhancing ways.
- Rational beliefs have a constructive impact on your subsequent thinking. Thus, they lead you to think realistically about yourself, others and the world. In particular, they help you to accept that good, bad and neutral things can result from the adversity that you are facing.

I have now introduced you to the core of REBT's view of psychological problems. If you are using this workbook in conjunction with consulting an REBT therapist or counsellor and you have any questions about REBT's view of psychological problems, ask your therapist to answer your questions. His or her answers will help you to determine whether or not REBT's view of psychological problems makes sense of your own problems for which you are seeking help.

If you are using this workbook as a self-help guide independently of seeing an REBT therapist, then I will now try to anticipate some of your questions about REBT's view of psychological problems by listing and answering some of the most commonly asked questions about this view.

Commonly asked questions about REBT's view of psychological problems

Question 1 Isn't the idea that psychological problems are caused by irrational beliefs overly simplistic?

Response First, I have not claimed that psychological problems are caused by irrational beliefs, nor I have said that irrational beliefs are the only factors to be taken into account when making sense of these problems. What I am saying is that of all the factors that are involved in these problems, irrational beliefs are at the core of them, meaning that according to REBT, they are the most important determining factor.

Question 2 But surely some highly aversive events like being raped or seeing a loved one murdered cause psychological problems. By saying that irrational beliefs are at the core of these problems, aren't you making light of such events?

Response You are making two points here which I will consider separately. First, you are claiming that highly aversive events cause psychological problems. Well, fortunately this isn't the case. What is true is that virtually all humans generally respond to such events with distress (or what we in REBT refer to as healthy negative emotions). This distress can be acute, but is based on healthy thinking. It is also true that many people respond to these events with disturbance (or what we in REBT refer to as unhealthy negative emotions). Such disturbance can also be acute and is based on unhealthy thinking. Now, in many of the latter cases, these disturbed reactions are short-lived and do not warrant the services of a therapist. REBT therapists would only intervene when the person concerned has become 'stuck', as it were, in this disturbed response mode and in doing so, we usually find that the person has become stuck in viewing the event through the lenses of an irrational belief. Once we have helped the person think rationally about the highly aversive event, he or she can feel healthily distressed about it and experiencing these healthy negative feelings helps the person go through the healing process.

This response has paved the way for me to address your second point which is that saying that irrational beliefs are at the core of a 'sustained' (my addition) disturbed response to a highly aversive event makes light of this event. I would dispute this. As I have said, as an REBT therapist I would only intervene in using REBT with a person when that person has become stuck in a disturbed response mode about the highly aversive event. My initial goal in intervening in this way would be to help the person experience strong feelings of healthy distress about the event and in doing this I am, in effect, saying that the event is highly aversive. If I were aiming to encourage the person to feel nothing or to feel mild feelings of distress then I would be guilty of making light of this event, but as I have said this is not my goal. Thus, I and other REBT therapists are not guilty of this charge.

Question 3 Aren't there certain things in life that we humans must have, like being loved and having control over our lives?

Response My answer to this question is a resounding 'no', if you are speaking about adults and if you mean that all humans are bound to be psychologically disturbed if we aren't loved or don't have control over our lives. Now, I do concede that being loved and having control over our lives are important human desires and we are far happier when we are loved and have control over our lives than when we are not. But this doesn't mean that being loved and having control are absolute necessities and that psychological problems are inevitable consequences of their absence. If this were true then all humans would have to have psychological problems when we weren't loved or didn't have control over our lives *no matter what we believed about their absence from our lives*, and we know that this isn't true. There is only one situation to which all humans would respond with psychological disturbance – and this is sensory deprivation. But even here, there would be much variation with some humans becoming disturbed very quickly and others becoming so much later.

The REBT position is that as humans we have many desires and if we don't transform these into dire necessities then we won't experience psychological problems. We will, of course, experience healthy negative emotions when our desires aren't met. This position is the one that I illustrated when I took you through the 'Giving a Speech' model earlier in this chapter (see pp. 3–5).

Question 4 You imply that there is nothing awful in the world. What about the holocaust, wasn't that awful?

Response Here, you are referring to awfulizing beliefs (see p. 7). With respect to the holocaust, holding an awfulizing belief means, amongst other things, (a) that the holocaust absolutely should not have happened or absolutely should not have been as bad as it was, and (b) that no good could possibly have come from it. First, tragically, the holocaust did happen and it was as bad as it was. On that score, the awfulizing belief is false. Second, we know that good did come from the holocaust. It is unlikely that the State of Israel would have been founded as soon after the war if it wasn't for the holocaust, so again this falsifies the awfulizing belief. Now, saying that it was not awful that the holocaust happened does not in any shape or form mean that it was not a truly tragic catastrophe. It means that sadly we have to accept that we live in a world where such catastrophes can and do happen and thanks to the indomitability of the human spirit we can transcend such catastrophes and move on with our lives.

You may think that I am playing with words here, but I am not. I am distinguishing between 'awful' which does not exist and catastrophes which, sadly, do exist.

Question 5 Doesn't the principle of acceptance encourage complacency?

Response No, it does not. Let me explain my answer with respect to self-acceptance. If you accept yourself for giving a poor speech, for example, you are saying that (a) you are a fallible human being who is capable of performing well, poorly and neutrally and cannot be defined by giving a poor speech and that (b) the speech that you gave was poor and you can improve. If giving a good speech is important to you, accepting yourself will help you to reflect on the reasons why you gave a poor speech and motivate you to improve your performance in the future. This is the antithesis of complacency which means that you have no incentive to improve your speech-making ability. Incidentally, depreciating yourself for giving a poor speech will not help you to improve your speech-making ability because instead of reflecting on the reasons why your speech was poor, you will be preoccupied with your ineptitude as a person.

Question 6 You've said nothing about the past. What is REBT's view about the role of the past in psychological problems?

Response Although REBT is known as a present-centred and future-oriented approach to psychotherapy, it does not neglect a person's past at all. It does not argue, however, that your past experiences cause your present psychological problems. Rather, it holds that your past contributes to these problems – an important difference. Let me explain what I mean by this.

Let's suppose that your parents neglected you when you were growing up and you blame them for causing your present feelings of depression. This is an understandable reaction on your part, but an incorrect one. Would a hundred people of your age, gender and intelligence, who were exposed to the same level of parental neglect all feel depressed about it now? Hardly! A lot would, I grant you, feel depressed about it, but some would feel sad and some would even feel glad, arguing that it helped them to stand on their own two feet. This echoes REBT's reformulation of Epictetus' dictum which, when applied to the past reads:

> People are disturbed, not by events in their past, but by their rigid and extreme views of these events.

Having said this, REBT does not deny that your past has some influence on your present feelings. It would certainly agree that it would have been better for you then and now, if your parents had not neglected you, but showed you due care and attention instead. It would argue that feelings of sadness would be a healthy response to this neglect since it would be based on a full preference and not on a demand. If it mattered to you that your parents neglected you (as it would to most, but not all, people), it would hardly be healthy for you to feel happy or indifferent about this neglect. So your past, if you will, restricts your choice about the type of feelings you are likely to experience about parental neglect (in this case, negative rather than positive or neutral), but your beliefs (rational or irrational) determine whether your negative feelings about this neglect are likely to be healthy (rational beliefs) or unhealthy (irrational beliefs). Let me sum up REBT's view on this point with two equations:

Past neglect + irrational beliefs = depression
Past neglect + rational beliefs = sadness

Question 7 But in saying that my disturbed feelings are largely determined by my irrational beliefs, aren't you blaming me for having these disturbed feelings?

Response No, not at all. If I were blaming you, I would be saying, in effect, that you were a bad person for having disturbed feelings and the irrational beliefs that underpin them. And I am certainly not saying that. What I am saying is that you have responsibility for your disturbed feelings and the underpinning irrational beliefs. After all, they are your beliefs and no-one else's. If other people were responsible for the irrational beliefs that you hold, we would have to bring them into therapy and have them change which is a ridiculous notion. So, in REBT we hold you responsible for the beliefs that you hold and the feelings that you thereby create without blaming you. This is a liberating message because it states that you can change how you feel by changing the beliefs that you hold. You don't have to rely on changing others or situations first, which, if this was the case, would make personal change very much more difficult.

I have now outlined the REBT view of psychological problems and dealt with the most common questions that people ask about this view. I hope that you have sufficient information about the REBT view on this issue to consent to proceed to the next chapter in which I will outline the main principles of the practice of REBT.

Chapter 2

The practice of REBT

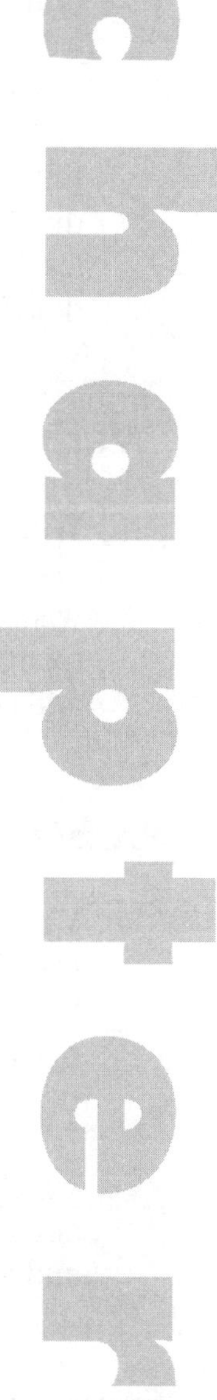

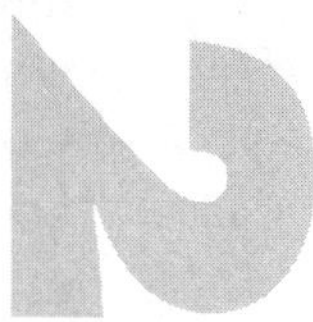

In this chapter, I am going to outline some of the major principles of REBT practice. In doing so I am writing primarily for those of you who are using this workbook on your own as a self-help guide, and thus, I will concentrate on the nature of 'workbook-delivered' REBT and the tasks that it calls upon you to perform. I will then write more generally about 'therapist-delivered' REBT, filling in some of the blanks about the practice of REBT that I haven't discussed in the former section. In addition, those of you who are consulting an REBT practitioner should preferably discuss the nature of 'therapist-delivered' REBT with your therapist.

'Workbook-delivered' REBT

What I call 'workbook-delivered' REBT has a number of distinguishing features. I will discuss these features to help you decide whether or not you wish to proceed further with this workbook which contains many practical exercises for you to engage in to help you to solve your emotional problems and achieve your goals.

Problem-focused and goal-oriented approach

Workbook-delivered REBT encourages you to specify your psychological problems one by one and to specify what you consider to be realistic goals for each of your problems. It also encourages you to focus on your problems one at a time, as far as this is practical, and to work steadily towards your goals. It is thus problem-focused and goal-oriented.

These two emphases are also a feature of 'therapist-delivered' REBT which contrasts sharply with some other counselling approaches that encourage you to discuss anything that you wish to discuss in an open-ended manner and do not adopt a goal-oriented stance.

Structured and logical approach

Workbook-delivered REBT is structured in nature and presented in a logical order. First, let me discuss its structured nature. If you were to consult a therapist from the psychodynamic or person-centred schools, you would discover that these therapists would encourage you to discuss and explore whatever you wanted and would provide little overt structure in which you would be expected to work. Given the lack of structure inherent in these approaches, it is difficult to imagine them spawning workbooks that are, in general, structured. So, if you are looking for a therapeutic experience in which you can explore whatever you want to, in whichever way you want, then this workbook is not for you and REBT is also probably not for you. However, if you are looking for a structured approach to emotional problem solving in which you are offered (a) a structured framework based on the REBT view of psychological problems (outlined in Chapter 1) for understanding the factors that are at the core of your problems, and (b) a structured way of dealing with these factors, then this workbook in particular, and REBT in general, are likely to be helpful to you.

Second, workbook-delivered REBT is logical in that you are offered a sensible, understandable step-by-step approach to solving your psychological problems where one step follows on logically from the previous step.

Educational approach

REBT is an educational approach to counselling and psychotherapy. This is demonstrated in several different ways in this workbook.

1 It teaches the REBT view of psychological problems (see Chapter 1).
2 It teaches a framework for assessing your problems and in particular for identifying the irrational beliefs that underpin these problems.
3 It shows you quite specifically how to question these irrational beliefs and their rational alternatives so that you can clearly see why your irrational beliefs are inconsistent with reality, illogical and detrimental to your mental health and to your interpersonal relationships, and why, by contrast, your rational beliefs are consistent with reality, logical and conducive to your mental health and your relationships with others.
4 It teaches you a variety of methods in step-by-step form to strengthen your conviction in your rational beliefs and to weaken your conviction in your irrational beliefs.
5 Throughout, it helps you to identify your doubts, reservations and objections to what is being presented to you, and helps you to evaluate them in a realistic way.
6 It helps you to understand the process of belief change so that you can foresee what is likely to happen when you try to change enduring irrational beliefs.
7 It helps you to identify and deal with factors that might otherwise lead to relapse.
8 It helps you to identify and surmount a host of obstacles to personal change.

Directive approach

Throughout this workbook I will direct your attention to factors considered by REBT to be important if you are to assess your problems accurately and to overcome them successfully. In this sense workbook-delivered REBT is directive in nature. Let me give you a flavour of what I will direct you to. Early in the process I will direct you as follows.

1 To consider the nature of your problems and to set a realistic goal for each of these problems.
2 To select a problem that you wish to tackle first (this problem is known as a target problem) and to choose a specific example of this problem to work on. Working with a specific example of your target problem allows me to direct you to identify:

 a) your most disturbed feeling and how you acted or felt like acting when you felt that way;
 b) what you were most disturbed about in this episode (known as the critical *A*);
 c) what specific irrational beliefs you held about this critical *A* that were at the core of your disturbed emotion and behaviour and what would be healthy alternatives to these rational beliefs;
 d) what would be a more constructive way of handling this situation.

Then I will direct you:

 e) to question your irrational and rational beliefs so that you can see why your irrational beliefs are irrational and why your rational beliefs are rational;
 f) to identify and respond constructively to any doubts, reservations or objections you have about your goals and what you need to do to achieve them; and
 g) to see what you need to do to strengthen your conviction in your rational beliefs and to weaken your conviction in your irrational beliefs so that you can achieve your goals.

Primarily present-centred and future-oriented approach

REBT is primarily a present-centred and future-oriented approach to psychotherapy and this is reflected in this workbook. However, this does not mean that you cannot look back and deal with your present feelings about past experiences or even your past feelings about past experiences. Just because REBT has a particular emphasis does not mean that other emphases are excluded altogether. So feel free to work on any problem, past, present and anticipated in this workbook.

Skills-focused approach

One of the features of this workbook is that it is skills-focused as is the wider practice of REBT. This means that in this workbook I will attempt to help you by teaching you in a step-by-step manner the skills of REBT self-help therapy. There is an adage in the field of counselling and psychotherapy which states that effective therapy is based on effective self-therapy. This is particularly true for a technically oriented approach such as REBT. In a skills-focused approach I:

1 teach you the skills of REBT, one at a time;
2 provide you with a worked example of each skill (with examples from actual clients who have given permission for their work to be presented here with light editing for easier reading and with appropriate comment from me);
3 give you an opportunity to practise the skills;
4 alert you to possible difficulties you might face implementing the skills and help you to minimize these difficulties; and
5 encourage you to practise the skills regularly during the week. Here, I recommend thirty minutes a day practice (equivalent to one episode of East Enders or Coronation Street). As I will reiterate throughout this workbook, unless you practise these skills, you will not internalize them.

If you are using this guide in conjunction with seeing an REBT therapist, you will get feedback on your skills from your therapist that is individually tailored. If you are working alone, this individually tailored feedback will not be available to you and this again is a drawback of using workbook-delivered REBT on your own. However, since I will be alerting you to common errors that clients make while learning the skills of REBT, I am hoping to cover at least some of the mistakes that you are likely to make.

'Therapist-delivered' REBT

'Therapist-delivered' REBT has the same emphases as workbook-delivered REBT. Thus, it is structured and logical, educational, directive, primarily present-centred and future-oriented and skills-focused. However, because therapist-delivered REBT is an interactive experience, your therapist may depart at times from these emphases to provide you with a 'bespoke' approach to therapy (i.e. an approach that is individually tailored to your therapeutic requirements). One might say that while 'workbook-delivered' REBT is 'off-the-peg' therapy, therapist-delivered REBT is 'made-to-measure' therapy. For example, there may be times during therapist-delivered REBT when it would be useful for you to talk in an unstructured way about your past experiences. A sensitive REBT practitioner would enable you to do this without structuring your exploration in any way or without directing you to your underlying irrational beliefs. There may be other times when taking a short break from the skills-based nature of REBT would be useful and again a flexible REBT therapist would allow you to do this.

So, if you are using this workbook in conjunction with seeing an REBT therapist, there may be occasions when you won't be using this workbook. Paradoxically, then, good REBT therapists don't always practise structured and logical, educationally based, directive, present or future-oriented, skills-focused REBT. They primarily do so, of course, otherwise they would not be REBT therapists, but there will be times when they do not. If you are consulting an REBT therapist, don't hesitate to discuss with him or her your wish to depart at times from traditional REBT, as we may call it.

It is in the nature of workbook-delivered REBT, where you are working alone with the workbook as your guide, that this level of flexibility is absent. This is a drawback of any workbook-delivered therapy and as such it is important that you accept this limitation while you work your way through the exercises in the forthcoming chapters. Before you proceed, let me first consider some of the most commonly asked questions 'applicants' have about the practice of REBT (workbook-delivered and therapist-delivered) before I get down to the nitty-gritty of helping you with your problems.

Commonly asked questions about the practice of REBT

Question 1 The way you describe it, REBT sounds like brainwashing. Am I right?

Response No, you're wrong. Brainwashing is a process that would involve you being taken away from your normal environment and deprived of food and sleep until you are susceptible to believing what the 'brainwasher' wants you to believe. In short, it is a process in which you are placed in a situation in which you are unable to use your critical faculties. In contrast, REBT is a process in which you are encouraged to:

1 use your critical faculties about the REBT view of psychological problems and the practice of REBT;
2 ask critical questions which are answered openly and honestly (honesty and openness are not noted characteristics of the brainwasher!);

3 voice your doubts, reservations or objections about what you are learning.

You are offered a definite framework in which to work in REBT, but in no shape or form are you compelled to use it or forced to suspend critical belief. Thus, REBT is almost the polar opposite of brainwashing.

Question 2 But aren't you telling me what to feel and what to do?

Response No, I'm neither telling you what to feel nor what to do. Let's take the issue of emotion first. In REBT we distinguish between healthy and unhealthy negative emotional responses to negative events. We certainly help you to see what the healthy alternative to a disturbed emotion is, but hardly tell you that you have to feel that way. In other words, we spell out what your feeling options are and encourage you to choose a response that is in your long-term healthy interests. If you select an emotional response that we do not consider to be in your long-term healthy interests, we may well express this reservation and explain why we have it. But this is very different from telling you what to feel.

Moving on to the issue of behaviour, in REBT we don't tell you what to do. Rather, we encourage you to act in ways that are consistent with your developing rational beliefs. Similarly, we don't tell you what not to do; rather, we discourage you from acting in ways that are consistent with your irrational beliefs. Put another way, once we have helped you to set goals that are in your healthy best interests, we help you to choose behaviours that will help you to realise these goals and to refrain from behaviours that prevent you from achieving them. This is very different from telling you what to do.

Question 3 Isn't it the case that REBT is only concerned with changing beliefs?

Response No. REBT is mainly concerned with helping you to change your beliefs, but as a means to an end. The end is a healthier way of responding emotionally and behaviourally to life's adversities. Having said this, REBT is also concerned to help you to develop a realistic view of the world free from a number of thinking distortions which affect the inferences that you make about events. In addition, REBT is concerned to help you to develop a range of interpersonal and problem-solving skills that will help you to become more effective in love, friendship and at work. Unfortunately, space constraints mean that I will not be able to highlight this aspect of REBT skills development, but it is very much a feature of ongoing therapist-delivered REBT.

Question 4 But how do I really change my beliefs?

Response This is an important question. From an REBT perspective, there are two major stages in belief change. In the first stage, you understand intellectually why your irrational beliefs are irrational and why your rational beliefs are rational. This is known as the stage of intellectual insight where your level of conviction in your rational belief affects your intellectual understanding, but is not sufficiently strong to influence for the better how you feel and act. Here you might say something like: 'Yes, I understand what you're saying (about a rational belief) in my head, but I don't really believe it in my gut'. What you are pointing to here is that you lack a level of insight associated with the second stage. This is known as emotional insight. Here your level of conviction in your rational belief is such that it influences for the better how you feel and how you act and you are able to say that you feel it is true in your gut. I will deal with the important issue of strengthening your conviction in your rational beliefs (and weakening your conviction in your irrational beliefs) in Chapter 12.

Question 5 I've read that the most important ingredient in psychotherapy is the relationship between therapist and client. Doesn't REBT neglect this relationship and overemphasize the importance of techniques?

Response The REBT position on the role of the therapist–client relationship in therapist-delivered psychotherapy is that it is an important ingredient in helping clients to change, but that it is neither necessary nor sufficient for such change to occur. Thus, if you are consulting an REBT therapist, it is important that you experience your therapist as empathic, respectful and genuine, but unless you identify, challenge and change your irrational beliefs, then you will not overcome your psychological problems. Having said this, experiencing your therapist as empathic, respectful and genuine may help you to identify, challenge and change your irrational beliefs and this is why I say that your relationship with your REBT therapist may be an important factor in helping you to overcome your problems. But having a good relationship with your therapist will not, on its own, help you to change.

Now, if you are using this workbook to help you to overcome your psychological problems without the help of a therapist, then you will not have the benefit of a therapeutic relationship to help you. This does not mean, however, that you cannot benefit from 'workbook-delivered' REBT. You can benefit if you follow the guidelines that I will be outlining and if you do so regularly and persistently. Whether this means that we 'overemphasize' the importance of techniques, I'm not sure. It does mean that our view is that unless you learn to become your own therapist and take responsibility for practising over time the techniques that I will teach you in this workbook, then you will not experience lasting change.

It's decision time

I have now discussed both the REBT view of psychological problems and its mode of practice and have answered some of the most commonly asked questions that people have about the theory and practice of this approach to therapy. You are now sufficiently informed about REBT to give your informed consent to proceed. If you are consulting an REBT therapist and you need further clarification on any of the points that I have raised, ask your therapist. But whether or not you are seeing an REBT therapist it's decision time. If you want to proceed, in the next chapter I will discuss the construction of a problem list and give guidance on how to set goals. If you decide to seek another therapeutic approach, good luck and thanks for considering REBT.

Chapter 3

Developing a problem list and setting goals

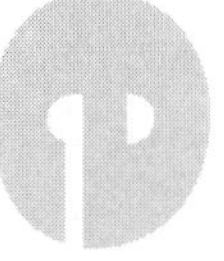
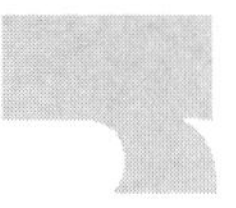
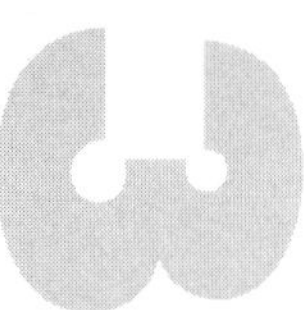

You have now given your informed consent to proceed with this workbook and are either using it on your own or in conjunction with seeing an REBT therapist. You are now ready to take the first step in dealing with your psychological problems. This step involves you specifying exactly which problems you wish to tackle. But first, let me discuss the elements of a psychological problem that we particularly look for in REBT.

Elements of a psychological problem

In the first half of this chapter I am going to show you what you need to do in order to develop a problem list. As the term suggests, this is a list of your psychological problems that you wish to tackle during the course of REBT. You may think that this will be quite easy for you, after all you know what your problems are. Well, in some cases it will be quite easy for you to develop a problem list, but in other cases you will encounter hidden pitfalls. In this section I will spell out and discuss the elements of a psychological problem that we particularly highlight in REBT. A psychological problem is one that:

1 *you* consider to be a problem for you and for which you are seeking help;
2 is about something that is either outside or within your orbit;
3 frequently involves the presence of a psychological theme;
4 usually involves you experiencing an unhealthy negative emotion;
5 usually involves you acting (or 'feeling like' acting) in ways that perpetuate the problem in the long term.

Let me consider each of these elements in greater detail.

You consider that your psychological problem is a problem for you and you are seeking help for this problem

At work you notice that a colleague experiences a great deal of anxiety about attending briefing meetings. Out of the goodness of your heart you buy them a copy of this workbook so that they can do something to overcome this problem. Your gift is first met with surprise and then irritation on the part of your colleague when it dawns on them why you bought the book because they don't think that they have a psychological problem. Although they may well be regularly anxious in the briefing meeting, for the present purposes, they don't have a problem unless they acknowledge that they have one. If you don't think you have a problem then you don't seek help. This is further demonstrated by the following.

On occasion, somebody telephones me to make an appointment for their spouse, close relative or offspring for counselling. My response is to suggest that the person concerned telephones me to make the appointment so that I know that they are requesting help. Even when this happens and I meet the person face to face, it sometimes transpires that they are only seeing me to please the other person and that they do not think that they have a psychological problem. They may, in fact, have a psychological problem as judged by textbooks on psychopathology, but unless they admit to having one, for the purposes of the workbook they don't have one that they are seeking help for.

So, only list psychological problems that you consider to be a problem for you and for which you are seeking help.

Your psychological problem is about something that emanates either from outside you or from within you

When you are feeling psychologically disturbed your feelings are about something that emanates either from outside of you and is thus largely outside your control or from within you and thus within your control to a greater or lesser extent. What is external to you (and thus largely outside your control) are other people's behaviour or lack of behaviour, specific events that are not authored by you, and more general environmental contexts. All these clearly emanate from outside you and are outside of your control even though some of them may be influenced by you. Thus, while you may be able to influence the way another person acts, in the final analysis the way that person behaves is beyond your control because the other person is separate from you and external to you. In REBT we call such events *external activating events*.

What is within your control (although not perfectly so) are events that emanate from within you such as your behaviour or lack of behaviour, your feelings, sensations, thoughts, images and everything to do with your physiological and other bodily responses. Even though all of these emanate from within you (and most are literally internal to you), it does not follow that you can control all of them. Thus, if you try to control the functioning of certain vital organs you cannot do so by an act of will, but the way in which you live your life can have an effect on those organs so you have control to this extent. Similarly, if you try to stop thinking certain thoughts, you will paradoxically increase the frequency of such thoughts, thus to gain control you have to allow yourself to think whatever you think, although even then your control will be far from complete. In REBT, we call such events *internal activating events*.

Your psychological problem frequently involves the presence of a psychological theme

When you examine closely what you are disturbed about it, it is likely that you will discover the presence of a particular psychological theme. Here is a partial list of common themes that feature in people's psychological problems:

failure	betrayal
rejection	unfairness
disapproval	illness
uncertainty	frustration
lack of control	criticism

Your psychological problem usually involves you experiencing an unhealthy negative emotion

Amongst other things, your emotions provide you with a readout concerning what is happening in your life. Thus, one way you know that you are experiencing a psychological problem is that your feelings tell you so.

I mentioned in Chapter 1 that REBT distinguishes between unhealthy negative emotions and healthy negative emotions. Usually you only experience the former when you have a psychological problem. How can you differentiate between a negative emotion that is unhealthy and one that is unhealthy? The following lists will help you.

An unhealthy negative emotion	*A healthy negative emotion*
Stems from an irrational belief	Stems from a rational belief
Leads to unconstructive behaviour	Leads to constructive behaviour
Interferes with constructive attempts to change the negative situation if it can be changed	Promotes constructive attempts to change the negative situation if it can be changed
Interferes with constructive adjustment if the negative situation cannot be changed	Promotes constructive adjustment if the negative situation cannot be changed
Leads to distorted thinking	Leads to realistic thinking
Interferes with problem solving	Promotes problem solving
Interferes with goal achievement	Aids goal achievement

The English language is not blessed with precise terms to help you to discriminate between unhealthy negative emotions and their healthy counterparts. Given this, I will outline the terms that I use in this workbook to describe unhealthy and healthy negative emotions, however if you find other terms more meaningful for you then use your own terms. The main point that you need to remember is that for every unhealthy negative emotion there is a healthy alternative. Now, let me list the terms that I will be using throughout this workbook. When you read these terms, keep in mind the features that differentiate between unhealthy and healthy negative emotions that I have just listed above.

Unhealthy negative emotion	*Healthy negative emotion*
Anxiety	Concern
Depression	Sadness
Guilt	Remorse
Shame	Disappointment
Hurt	Sorrow
Unhealthy anger	Healthy anger
Unhealthy jealousy	Healthy jealousy
Unhealthy envy	Healthy envy

One of the ways in which REBT differs from other approaches to psychotherapy lies in its approach to goal setting with respect to unhealthy negative emotions. Our goal when we help you to overcome your psychological problems is to help you to move from experiencing unhealthy negative emotions to healthy negative emotions in the face of negative life events and to do so at an equivalent level of intensity.

Let me explain what I mean by this. Imagine that you feel very anxious about the prospect of acting foolishly in public meetings at work and let's suppose that you rate the level of intensity of your anxiety at 85 per cent. To help you to overcome this psychological problem, I would help you to feel very concerned (at the equivalent 85 per cent level), but unanxious about this prospect. Since your feelings of anxiety stem from an irrational belief and your feelings of concern stem from a rational belief they are qualitatively different (because irrational beliefs and their rational equivalents are qualitatively different), these different feelings have to be on two continua as shown below.

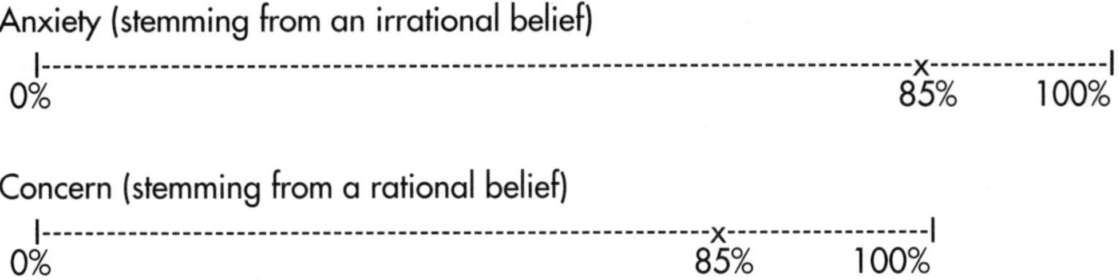

You will note from the length of these two continua that the maximum intensity of unhealthy negative emotions is greater than the maximum intensity of healthy negative emotions and this is particularly true for anxiety/concern and unhealthy anger/healthy anger. Given this, in REBT we strive to help you to achieve the *equivalent* level of intensity. It is important for you to grasp that we don't help you to feel less anxious (because this would mean that you would still hold an irrational belief, albeit with less conviction), nor do we help you to reduce your level of concern. A level of 85 per cent of concern indicates that you hold a strong rational belief and there is nothing unhealthy about doing so. If we were to help you to reduce your level of concern, we would in effect be helping you to lie to yourself and encouraging you to persuade yourself that your healthy flexible preference about not acting foolishly in public is less strong than it actually is.

Your psychological problem usually involves you acting (or 'feeling like' acting) in ways that perpetuate the problem in the long term

When you have a psychological problem, you not only experience an unhealthy negative emotion, you also act or 'feel like' acting in an unconstructive manner. Such unconstructive behaviour can take a number of different forms. Thus, your problem-related behaviour can:

1. be consistent with your unhealthy negative emotion (e.g. when you attack someone verbally towards whom you feel unhealthily angry);
2. help you to rid yourself of the unhealthy negative emotion once you have started to experience it (e.g. when you seek reassurance from someone when you begin to feel anxious about something);
3. help prevent you from feeling an unhealthy negative emotion (e.g. when you avoid a situation in which you would otherwise feel anxious were you to face it);
4. help you to compensate for the irrational belief that underpins your unhealthy negative emotion (e.g. when you try to show yourself how strong you are when you privately think that you are a weak person).

It is important for you to remember that whatever purpose your problem-related behaviour has, its effect is usually to perpetuate your psychological problem. This is why we help you not only to change your irrational beliefs in REBT, but also to change your behaviour so that you act in ways that are consistent with your developing rational beliefs.

Developing a problem list

A problem list is exactly what it says it is – a list of problems. This is what you do when you identify one of your psychological problems.

1 Think of the situations in which you experience the problem, e.g. '*speaking in public*'.
2 Identify the theme of the problem, what it is about the situations that you specified that is a problem for you. You may have already expressed the theme of the problem in step 1, e.g '*acting foolishly*'.
3 Identify the one major unhealthy emotion from the list below that you experience when you encounter the situations or themes specified above, you may experience several unhealthy emotions, but select the main *one*, e.g. anxiety.

Anxiety	Hurt
Depression	Unhealthy anger
Guilt	Unhealthy jealousy
Shame	Unhealthy envy

4 Identify the relevant behaviour that is related to the problem, e.g. 'to cope with my anxiety, I overprepare my material'.

The next stage is to put all the elements together in a sentence. Let me show you how to do this by first placing each element under its relevant heading.

Type of situation	*Theme*	*Unhealthy negative emotion*	*Behaviour*
When I have to speak in public	I think I might act foolishly	I feel anxious	To cope with my anxiety I over-prepare my material

Now, here is the sentence:

> When I have to speak in public and think that I might act foolishly, I feel anxious and cope with my anxiety by overpreparing my material.

This then constitutes your problem.

Here are some other examples of problems. See if you can place each of the different elements under the appropriate heading.

1 'Whenever I am stuck in a traffic jam and blocked from achieving my goals I feel unhealthily angry and shout obscenities'.
2 'Whenever my mother criticizes me I think that I have done something wrong and feel guilty. I then beg her for forgiveness'.

3 'When I see my friends with their babies I focus on the fact that I don't have what they have and I feel unhealthily envious. When I feel this way I drink to blot out my feelings'.
4 'When I begin to feel anxious I think that I am beginning to lose control and become more anxious. Then I do whatever I can to gain an immediate sense of control'.
5 'When my friends don't phone me when they say they will I take this as a sign they don't care about me. I feel hurt about this and withdraw from them and other people'.
6 'Whenever I think that I have acted foolishly in public I feel ashamed and avoid meeting these people again' (note that the theme of the problem and the type of situation is the same in this identified problem).

Now use this format to develop your own list of problems. You might find it helpful to use Figure 3.1 for your problem list.

I have used Figure 3.2 to list the examples of problems given above.

Taking your problems and setting realistic goals

Once you have developed your problem list the next step is for you to set realistic goals with respect to each of your problems. This involves the following steps.

1 *Keep the type of situation in which you disturb yourself the same.* After all, it is possible that you may well encounter such situations in the future.
2 *Keep the theme about which you disturbed yourself the same.* Again it is possible that you may encounter situations in which the theme reflects reality. You will have an opportunity later to consider whether or not the theme is an accurate representation of reality.
3 *Change your unhealthy negative emotion to a healthy negative emotion.* This step is important in that it helps you to deal with negative situations in a healthy, but realistic way.
4 *Change your unconstructive behaviour to constructive behaviour.* Again, this step is important in that it helps you to act constructively in the face of negative situations.

Let me exemplify this goal-setting process by returning to the problem that I defined above. Let me first give the problem in sentence format.

> When I have to speak in public and think that I might act foolishly, I feel anxious and cope with my anxiety by overpreparing my material.

List your problems below

1
2
3
4
5
6

Figure 3.1 Problem list.

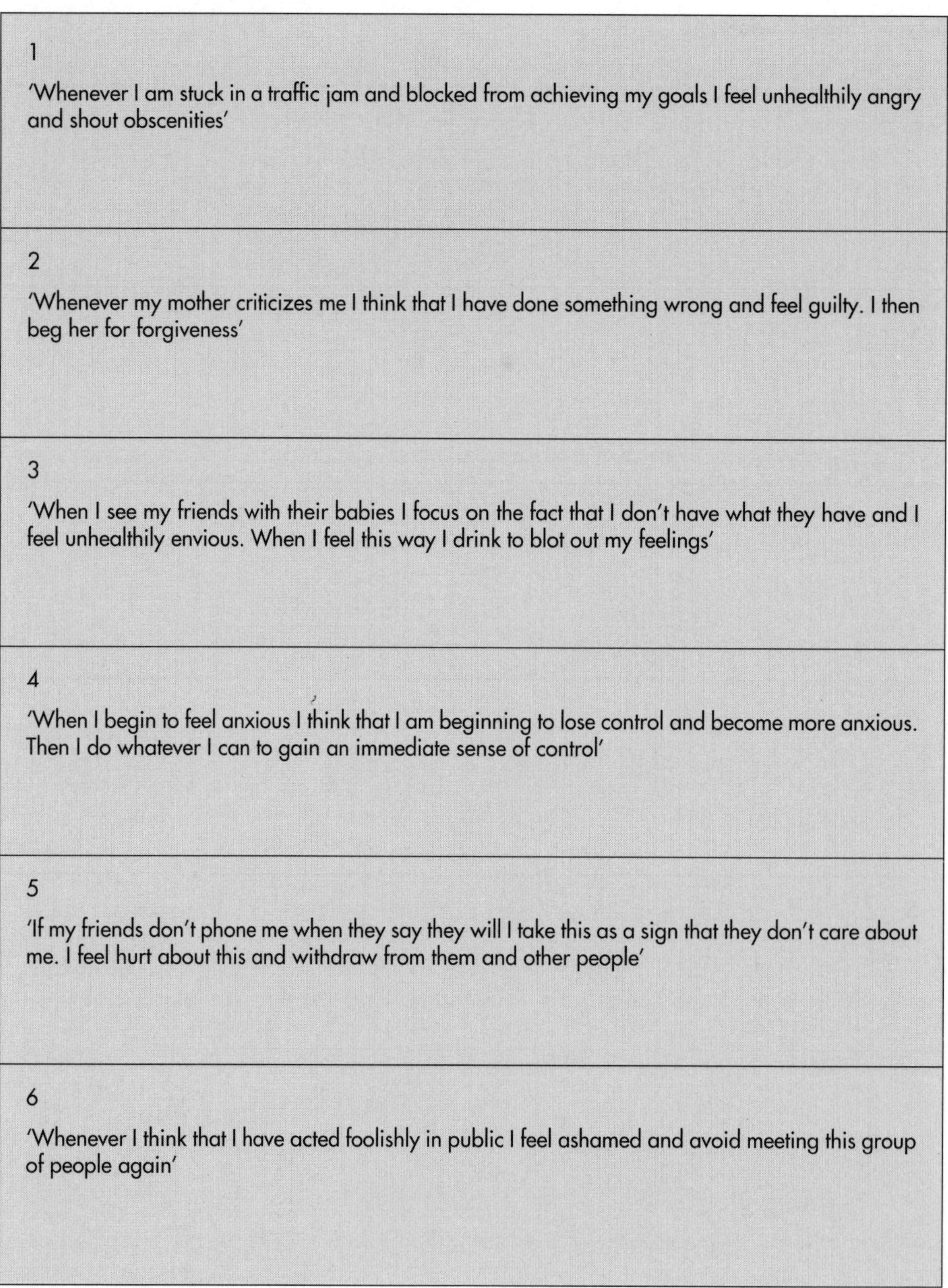

1

'Whenever I am stuck in a traffic jam and blocked from achieving my goals I feel unhealthily angry and shout obscenities'

2

'Whenever my mother criticizes me I think that I have done something wrong and feel guilty. I then beg her for forgiveness'

3

'When I see my friends with their babies I focus on the fact that I don't have what they have and I feel unhealthily envious. When I feel this way I drink to blot out my feelings'

4

'When I begin to feel anxious I think that I am beginning to lose control and become more anxious. Then I do whatever I can to gain an immediate sense of control'

5

'If my friends don't phone me when they say they will I take this as a sign that they don't care about me. I feel hurt about this and withdraw from them and other people'

6

'Whenever I think that I have acted foolishly in public I feel ashamed and avoid meeting this group of people again'

Figure 3.2 Problem list – examples.

Now let me present this problem element by element under the appropriate heading.

Type of situation	*Theme*	*Unhealthy negative emotion*	*Behaviour*
When I have to speak in public	I think I might act foolishly	I feel anxious	To cope with my anxiety I overprepare my material

If you follow the four guidelines that I outlined above you will note that in specifying your goal the first two elements are the same as in the defined problem.

Type of situation	*Theme*
When I have to speak in public	I think I might act foolishly

So all we have to do is to set goals with respect to emotion and behaviour. Let's do this one step at a time. First let's consider the emotional goal.

Type of situation	*Theme*	*Healthy negative emotion*
When I have to speak in public	I think I might act foolishly	I want to feel concern rather than anxiety

Here the person has correctly realized that the healthy emotional alternative to anxiety is concern. You will also note that the person has stated that his goal is concern *rather than* anxiety. I recommend using the phrase *rather than* because it will help you to differentiate between the healthy negative emotion (your goal) and the unhealthy negative emotion (your problem).

Now let's move on to the behavioural goal:

Type of situation	*Theme*	*Healthy negative emotion*	*Behaviour*
When I have to speak in public	I think I might act foolishly	I want to feel concern rather than anxiety	I want to prepare normally rather than overprepare my material

Again note that the person has stated that his goal is to prepare normally *rather than* to overprepare his material.

Below I have listed the goals with respect to each of the problems listed above. Again see if you can place each of the different elements under the appropriate heading.

1 'Whenever I am stuck in a traffic jam and blocked from achieving my goals, my goal is to feel healthily angry rather than unhealthily angry, and to keep my mouth shut and my mind on accepting that frustration is part of life rather than shouting obscenities'.
2 'Whenever my mother criticizes me and I think that I have done something wrong, my goal is to feel remorse rather than guilt and to apologize in an adult way rather than beg her for forgiveness'.
3 'When I see my friends with their babies and I focus on the fact that I don't have what they have, my goal is to experience healthy envy rather than unhealthy envy and to remind myself in writing of what I do have in my life as well as what I don't have, rather than drinking to blot out my feelings'.
4 'When I begin to feel anxious and I think that I am beginning to lose control, my goal is to feel concern about losing control rather than anxiety about it, and to stay with my feelings so that I can gradually regain control rather than doing whatever I can to gain an immediate sense of control'.
5 'When my friends don't phone me when they say they will and I take this as a sign that they don't care about me, my goal is to feel sorrow about this rather than hurt, and to express my feelings to them rather than withdrawing from them and others'.
6 'Whenever I think that I have acted foolishly in public, my goal is to feel disappointed rather than ashamed and to meet the members of this group again with my head held high rather than avoiding them'.

Now use this format to develop your goals with respect to each of your problems. You might find it helpful to use Figure 3.3 for your list of goals. You will note that on this figure there are spaces for you to rate your progress towards your goals. This is important because it will help you to see the fruits of your labours and to identify obstacles to change if you aren't making progress towards your goals.

I have used Figure 3.4 to list the examples of goals given above.

You will note that your goal statements assume that the themes in the problem situations are true. Of course they may not be and later in this workbook I will show you how to question whether or not your themes are accurate representations of the situations in which you experience your problems. The REBT view is that this is best done *after* you have made some progress at challenging your irrational beliefs and with developing your rational beliefs.

List your goals and rate the progress you are making towards them. Do this by choosing a number between 0 and 10, where 0 represents no progress and 10 represents 100 per cent progress, and record the date.

1						
2						
3						
4						
5						
6						

Figure 3.3 List of goals.

List your goals and rate the progress you are making towards them. Do this by choosing a number between 0 and 10, where 0 represents no progress and 10 represents 100 per cent progress, and record the date.						
1 'Whenever I am stuck in a traffic jam and blocked from achieving my goals, my goal is to feel healthily angry rather than unhealthily angry, and to keep my mouth shut and my mind on accepting that frustration is part of life rather than shouting obscenities'	4/1/00 1	8/2/00 3	1/3/00 6	15/3/00 9		
2 'Whenever my mother criticizes me and I think that I have done something wrong, my goal is to feel remorse rather than guilt and to apologize in an adult way rather than beg her for forgiveness'						
3 'When I see my friends with their babies and I focus on the fact that I don't have what they have, my goal is to experience healthy envy rather than unhealthy envy and to remind myself in writing of what I do have in my life as well as what I don't have, rather than drinking to blot out my feelings'						
4 'When I begin to feel anxious and I think that I am beginning to lose control, my goal is to feel concern about losing control rather than anxiety about it and to stay with my feelings so that I can gradually regain control rather than doing whatever I can to gain an immediate sense of control'						
5 'When my friends don't phone me when they say they will and I take this as a sign that they don't care about me, my goal is to feel sorrow about this rather than hurt and to express my feelings to them rather than withdrawing from them and others'						
6 'Whenever I think that I have acted foolishly in public, my goal is to feel disappointed rather than ashamed and to meet the members of this group again with my head held high rather than avoiding them'						

Figure 3.4 List of goals – examples.

Setting goals for a time after you have overcome your problems

Many years ago I used to have a very bad stammer and regarded the prospect of talking to a group with great anxiety. If I had used the present mode of problem formulation, I would have said:

> Whenever I have to speak to a group I think that I may stammer. I feel anxious about this and will either find some way of getting out of giving the talk or will overprepare my material.

I would then have set the following goal:

> Whenever I have to speak to a group I think that I may stammer. My goal is to feel concerned about this rather than anxious about it and to give the talk with a normal amount of preparation rather than finding some way of getting out of giving the talk or overpreparing my material.

Although I knew nothing about REBT at the time I acted in a way that was consistent with the above behavioural goal. As a result two things happened. First, after a while I lost my anxiety about the prospect of stammering when I spoke to groups and felt healthily concerned about this possibility and second, I stammered far less when giving such talks and developed a sense of competence about public speaking at which I am, if I may say so, now quite adept.

I have related this personal story to highlight the difference between two goals:

1 the goal of overcoming a psychological problem about a negative situation (in my case to feel concerned about stammering in front of a group);
2 the goal of enhancing personal development (in my case to stammer less and to increase my competence and skill at public speaking).

The REBT position is that both sets of goals are important but that the best way of achieving personal development goals is by first achieving the goal of overcoming psychological problems. This is so important that I am going to repeat it.

> The best way of achieving personal development goals is by first achieving the goal of overcoming psychological problems.

If we apply this principle to the goals that I have listed in Figure 3.4 we have the following personal development goals.

Goal 1

Overcoming psychological problem goal 'Whenever I am stuck in a traffic jam and blocked from achieving my goals, my goal is to feel healthily angry rather than unhealthily angry, and to keep my mouth shut and my mind on accepting that frustration is part of life rather than shouting obscenities'.

Personal development goal 'To utilize my time effectively when I am stuck in a traffic jam'.

Goal 2

Overcoming psychological problem goal 'Whenever my mother criticizes me and I think that I have done something wrong, my goal is to feel remorse rather than guilt and to apologize in an adult way rather than beg her for forgiveness'.

Personal development goal 'To think objectively about criticisms from my mother. If she has a point I will apologize. If she hasn't I will express my views clearly and assertively'.

Goal 3

Overcoming psychological problem goal 'When I see my friends with their babies and I focus on the fact that I don't have what they have, my goal is to experience healthy envy rather than unhealthy envy and to remind myself of what I do have in my life as well as what I don't have, rather than drinking to blot out my feelings'.

Personal development goal 'To enjoy being with my friends when they have their babies with them'.

Goal 4

Overcoming psychological problem goal 'When I begin to feel anxious and I think that I am beginning to lose control, my goal is to feel concern about losing control rather than anxiety about it, and to stay with my feelings so that I can gradually regain control rather than doing whatever I can to gain an immediate sense of control'.

Personal development goal 'To see that anxiety is a sign that there is a threat on the horizon and to learn to deal with this threat more effectively, rather than fearing loss of control'.

Goal 5

Overcoming psychological problem goal 'When my friends don't phone me when they say they will and I take this as a sign that they don't care about me, my goal is to feel sorrow about this rather than hurt, and to express my feelings to them rather than withdrawing from them and others'.

Personal development goal 'To develop more honest relationships with friends whether they phone me or not'.

Goal 6

Overcoming psychological problem goal 'Whenever I think that I have acted foolishly in public, my goal is to feel disappointed rather than ashamed and to meet the members of this group again with my head held high rather than avoiding them'.

Personal development goal 'To develop greater social poise'.

It is important for you to realize that you may not achieve your personal development goals, but you don't know this until you commit yourself to the necessary action. Thus, even though I overcame my anxiety about stammering in front of other people and continued to give public presentations, I may neither have developed competence at public speaking nor have come to enjoy it. If becoming skilled at public speaking and enjoying this activity were my personal development goal, I would only have discovered whether or not I could have realized it by taking the necessary steps, i.e. by speaking in public many times. In doing so, I may have found that the best I could achieve was to be below average at public speaking and to tolerate this activity rather than to enjoy it. If so, I would have concluded that my skills and interests lay elsewhere.

Figure 3.5 summarizes the work that I have discussed in this chapter. It shows defined problems and both 'overcoming psychological problem' goals and 'personal development' goals for each of the problems I have discussed.

It is now time for you to list your problems and to set goals. When you do the latter, make sure that you set both overcoming psychological problems goals and personal development goals. Do this in Figure 3.6.

<table>
<tr><td colspan="7">List your goals and rate the progress you are making towards them. Do this by choosing a number between 0 and 10, where 0 represents no progress and 10 represents 100 per cent progress, and record the date.</td></tr>
<tr><td>Goal 1

Overcoming psychological problem goal
'Whenever I am stuck in a traffic jam and blocked from achieving my goals, my goal is to feel healthily angry rather than unhealthily angry, and to keep my mouth shut and my mind on accepting that frustration is part of life rather than shouting obscenities'

Personal development goal
'To utilize my time effectively when I am stuck in a traffic jam'</td><td>4/1/00
1

4/4/00
2</td><td>8/2/00
3

18/4/00
6</td><td>1/3/00
6

1/5/00
9</td><td>15/3/00
9

15/5/00
10</td><td></td><td></td></tr>
<tr><td>Goal 2

Overcoming psychological problem goal
'Whenever my mother criticizes me and I think that I have done something wrong, my goal is to feel remorse rather than guilt and to apologize in an adult way rather than beg her for forgiveness'

Personal development goal
'To think objectively about criticisms from my mother. If she has a point I will apologize. If she hasn't, I will express my views clearly and assertively'</td><td></td><td></td><td></td><td></td><td></td><td></td></tr>
<tr><td>Goal 3

Overcoming psychological problem goal
'When I see my friends with their babies and I focus on the fact that I don't have what they have, my goal is to experience healthy envy rather than unhealthy envy and to remind myself in writing of what I do have in my life as well as what I don't have, rather than drinking to blot out my feelings'

Personal development goal
'To enjoy being with my friends when they have their babies with them'</td><td></td><td></td><td></td><td></td><td></td><td></td></tr>
</table>

continued . . .

<table>
<tr><td>Goal 4

Overcoming psychological problem goal
'When I begin to feel anxious and I think that I am beginning to lose control, my goal is to feel concern about losing control rather than anxiety about it, and to stay with my feelings so that I can gradually regain control rather than doing whatever I can to gain an immediate sense of control'

Personal development goal
'To see that anxiety is a sign that there is a threat on the horizon and to l earn to deal with this threat more effectively, rather than fearing loss of control'</td><td></td><td></td><td></td><td></td><td></td><td></td></tr>
<tr><td>Goal 5

Overcoming psychological problem goal
'If my friends don't phone me when they say they will and I take this as a sign that they don't care about me, my goal is to feel sorrow about this rather than hurt, and to express my feelings to them rather than withdrawing from them and others'

Personal development goal
'To develop more honest relationships with friends whether they phone me or not'</td><td></td><td></td><td></td><td></td><td></td><td></td></tr>
<tr><td>Goal 6

Overcoming psychological problem goal
'Whenever I think that I have acted foolishly in public, my goal is to feel disappointed rather than ashamed and to meet the members of this group again with my head held high rather than avoiding them'

Personal development goal
'To develop greater social poise'</td><td></td><td></td><td></td><td></td><td></td><td></td></tr>
</table>

Figure 3.5 List of goals for overcoming psychological problems (OPP) and for personal development (PD) – examples.

List your goals and rate the progress you are making towards them. Do this by choosing a number between 0 and 10, where 0 represents no progress and 10 represents 100 per cent progress, and record the date.

Goal 1 *Overcoming psychological problem goal* *Personal development goal*						
Goal 2 *Overcoming psychological problem goal* *Personal development goal*						
Goal 3 *Overcoming psychological problem goal* *Personal development goal*						

Figure 3.6 List of goals for overcoming psychological problems and for personal development.

Chapter 4

Choosing a target problem and assessing a specific example

Once you have constructed a problem list and set goals for each problem, the next step is for you to select a problem from your problem list that you would like to tackle first. This might be:

1 the problem that you are most disturbed about;
2 the problem that is easiest to tackle;
3 the problem that is most pressing for you to tackle at the moment; or
4 the problem that you are likely to make progress on most quickly.

In making your decision, it is important to bear in mind that in using this workbook you are likely to spend some time working on this selected problem – which in REBT we term the *target problem*. So, choose carefully.

While I suggest that you begin with a problem from your problem list, you can apply the information in this chapter and those that follow to any episode of emotional disturbance, whether or not it is an example of a problem from your problem list. Bear this point in mind as you proceed.

Selecting a specific example of your target problem to assess

Once you have chosen your target problem, the next step is for you to select a specific example of this target problem. At the beginning of the REBT process we usually start at the specific level and move on to the general level later on the basis that most people find it easier to move from the specific to the general than vice versa. We also begin at the specific level because when you assess specific examples of target problems you are likely to get more valid information than if you attempt to assess more general problems.

What kind of specific example of your target problem should you select? There are several possibilities:

1 a current example of your target problem;
2 a very recent example of your target problem;
3 a typical example of your target problem;
4 a vivid example of your target problem; or
5 a possible future example of your target problem.

When you have selected a specific example of your target problem, use the first page of the Dryden REBT Form (DRF-2) to assess it (see Figure 4.1). The complete version of the DRF-2 can be found in Appendix 1. Also, don't forget you can use this page to assess an episode of emotional disturbance whether or not it is an example of a problem on your problem list.

The Dryden REBT form (DRF-2)

1. **Situation**: briefly describe a specific situation in which you disturbed yourself

2. ***C* (Consequences)**: identify your major unhealthy negative emotion in this episode, choose one from: anxiety, depression, shame, guilt, hurt, unhealthy anger, unhealthy jealousy and unhealthy envy. Also specify how you acted (or 'felt like' acting) in this situation

   i) Emotional consequences =

   ii) Behavioural consequences =

3. **Critical *A* (Activating event)**: identify the aspect of the situation that you were most disturbed about at *C*

4. ***B* (Beliefs)**: identify your irrational beliefs about *A* and list their rational alternatives

i) **Demand =**	i) **Full preference =**
ii) **Awfulizing belief =**	ii) **Anti-awfulizing belief =**
iii) **Low frustration tolerance belief =**	iii) **High frustration tolerance belief =**
iv) **Depreciation belief =**	iv) **Acceptance belief =**

Figure 4.1 Page 1 of the Dryden REBT form (DRF-2).

1. **Situation**: briefly describe a specific situation in which you disturbed yourself

Figure 4.2 Describe the situation in which you disturbed yourself

Step 1: describe the situation

The first step in assessing the specific example of your target problem (or an episode of emotional disturbance) is to describe the situation in which you felt disturbed. To do this, use step 1 of the DRF-2 (see Figure 4.2). It is important to be as factual as possible about the situation and describe it from a dispassionate perspective or as an objective jury would. In general, refrain from making any inferences in your description. As you will presently see inferences go beyond the observable data, they may be accurate or inaccurate but they need to be tested against the available information. If you just cannot keep inferences out of your description of the situation that's not a grave problem. Describe the situation as accurately as you can.

Throughout this chapter I will use the example of Oliver whose target problem was as follows:

> Whenever I am in the company of authorities, I think that they will criticize me and I become anxious. When this happens I try to find an excuse to withdraw from the situation.

Oliver chose to assess a recent specific example of this target problem that I will refer to throughout this and the following chapters. Oliver's description of the situation in which he disturbed himself is found in Figure 4.3. You will note that Oliver's statement 'I received a memo to see my boss at the end of the working day' is a description of the event in the sense that were Oliver to show us the memo we would be able to check that Oliver's boss is, in fact, asking to see him at the end of the day. Even if the boss's request were made on the phone, Oliver's statement would still be a description of the situation because if we had listened to the call we would agree that Oliver's boss had acted in the way described by Oliver.

Let's suppose that Oliver had written instead 'I received a *harsh* memo from my boss to see him at the end of the day. *This means that I have done something wrong and he wants to criticize me*' as a description of the event. Would this still be a description of the situation in which Oliver felt disturbed? The answer would be a resounding 'No'.

1. **Situation**: briefly describe a specific situation in which you disturbed yourself

   I received a memo to see my boss at the end of the working day.

Figure 4.3 Oliver's description of the situation in his selected specific example of his target problem.

The parts of Oliver's statement that are in italics go beyond the data at hand and therefore constitute inferences about the situation rather than a description of it. The statement I have just attributed to Oliver includes two inferences which I will consider one at a time:

1 *harsh.*

Here, Oliver has inferred that the tone of his boss's voice was harsh. This is an inference because it represents Oliver's opinion about the tone of the memo. If, however, most objective people reading the memo agree with Oliver that the tone was harsh then we can say that by consensus the statement 'harsh memo' can be given the status of a description.

2 *This means that I have done something wrong and he wants to criticize me.*

Here, Oliver is clearly going well beyond the available information in claiming that his statement is part of the description of the situation that he was facing. All he knows at this point is that his boss wants to see him at the end of the day. He doesn't know why, he only knows when. His attempt to answer the question is thus an inference and is likely to reveal aspects of his psychological problem, for example that he may have a problem dealing with criticism.

In summary, when describing the situation refrain as far as you can from making any inferences that go beyond the information at hand.

Step 2: identify *C* – emotional and behavioural responses

The most common way that you are likely to know that you are experiencing a psychological problem is by the way that you feel and the way that you behave. Consequently, after you have described the situation in which you experienced the problem, the next step is to identify how you felt and/or acted (or 'felt like' acting) in that situation (see Figure 4.4)

Let's take a closer look at what you are called upon to do in step 2.

2. ***C* (Consequences)**: identify your major unhealthy negative emotion in this episode, choose one from: anxiety, depression, shame, guilt, hurt, unhealthy anger, unhealthy jealousy and unhealthy envy. Also specify how you acted (or 'felt like' acting) in this situation

   i) Emotional consequences =

   ii) Behavioural consequences =

Figure 4.4 Identify *C*.

Identify your major unhealthy negative emotion in this episode

If you go back to the target problem you will see that it contains an unhealthy negative emotion. Thus, this unhealthy negative emotion should also be the major unhealthy negative emotion that you experienced in the specific example of your target problem.

If not, choose a specific example where this emotion predominated and put this emotion in the appropriate space in Figure 4.4.

If you are assessing an episode of emotional disturbance that is not a specific example of a problem on your problem list then your major unhealthy negative emotion may not be so apparent. Indeed, in this episode you may have experienced a number of emotions. You may have experienced a number of unhealthy negative emotions and a number of healthy negative emotions. In step 2 you are being asked to identify *one* emotion. This emotion has to be an unhealthy negative emotion and it has to be the major one that you experienced (the emotion that lies at the core of your psychological problem). If you want to work on a second unhealthy negative emotion in this episode you will have to use a second DRF-2 form because it is very likely that what you are anxious about in a situation, for example, is likely to be different from what you are guilty about in that same situation. Also, you have not yet developed sufficient competence at using this form to be able to improvise successfully by accurately assessing two different unhealthy negative emotions at the same time. Using REBT on your problems is like playing jazz. Before you can improvise to good effect you need to become competent at the basic techniques.

You will see from the left hand column in Table 4.1 that I have provided a list of the unhealthy negative emotions that people frequently bring to counselling. I have already considered the issue of unhealthy negative

Table 4.1 Unhealthy and healthy negative emotions.

Unhealthy negative emotion	*Healthy negative emotion*
Anxiety	Concern
Depression	Sadness
Guilt	Remorse
Shame	Disappointment
Hurt	Sorrow
Unhealthy anger	Healthy anger
Unhealthy jealousy	Healthy jealousy
Unhealthy envy	Healthy envy

emotions in Chapter 3. Here it is important that you are not constrained by the terms that I have used in Table 4.1. Thus, if you tend to use the term 'rage' for unhealthy anger then feel free to use this term since it fits well with your experience.

Some of you may find it difficult to discriminate among the different unhealthy negative emotions. There are three ways in which you can do this:

- by considering what I call the major inference theme related to your unhealthy negative emotion;
- by considering the major actions and/or action tendencies related to each unhealthy negative emotion;
- by considering how you think or tend to think *after* you began to experience the unhealthy negative emotion.

Identify the major inference theme associated with your major unhealthy negative emotion

Table 4.2 lists the major inference themes that are related to the eight unhealthy negative emotions that regularly crop up in counselling. If you are unsure about which unhealthy negative emotion you *mainly* experienced in the specific example that you selected, consult this table and choose the inference theme that most closely reflects what you were disturbed about. Once you have done so, move to the left-hand column and look at the unhealthy negative emotion (UNE) that is related to your chosen inference theme. This is, in all probability, your major UNE.

Table 4.2 Inferential themes in unhealthy negative emotions.

Emotion	*Inferential themes*
Anxiety	Threat, danger
Depression	Loss, loss of value, failure
Shame	Public disclosure of weakness, falling very short of one's ideal
Guilt	Moral violation (sin of commission and omission), hurting others
Hurt	Others treat you badly (and you consider that you do not deserve such treatment)
Anger	Frustrated, transgressed against
Jealousy	Threat to present relationship posed by another person
Envy	Others experience the good fortune which you lack and covet

Identify the major action or tendency associated with your major unhealthy negative emotion

Here is a second way of identifying your major UNE. Table 4.3 lists the major actions and action tendencies (i.e. what you 'felt like' doing in the situation even if you didn't do it) associated with each unhealthy negative emotion and each healthy negative emotion. Choose the action or action tendency (in the right-hand column) that best reflects what you did or 'felt like' doing in the situation under consideration. Then move to the left-hand column and look at the negative emotion that is most closely related to your chosen action or action tendency. If the negative emotion is unhealthy this is, in all probability, your major UNE. If the negative emotion is healthy then you may have responded constructively in the situation which may, in retrospect, not be a good specific example of emotional disturbance.

Identify the way you thought after you began to experience your major unhealthy negative emotion

The third way of identifying your major UNE involves considering how you thought after you began to experience the emotion that you felt in the situation under consideration. Table 4.4 lists the major thinking consequences associated with each unhealthy negative emotion and each healthy negative emotion. Choose the type of thinking (in the right-hand column) that best reflects what you thought after you began to feel the emotion that you decided was the *major* one that you experienced in the situation under consideration. Then move to the left-hand column and look at the negative emotion that is

Table 4.3 Actions and action tendencies associated with unhealthy and healthy negative emotions.

Negative emotions	*Type*	*Action/action tendency*
Anxiety	Unhealthy	Avoiding threat, seeking reassurance even though you are not reassurable
Concern	Healthy	Confronting threat, seeking reassurance only when reassurable
Depression	Unhealthy	Prolonged withdrawal from enjoyable activities
Sadness	Healthy	Engagement with enjoyable activities after a period of mourning
Guilt	Unhealthy	Begging for forgiveness
Remorse	Healthy	Asking for forgiveness
Hurt	Unhealthy	Sulking
Sorrow	Healthy	Assertion
Shame	Unhealthy	Averting one's eyes from the gaze of others, withdrawal from others
Disappointment	Healthy	Maintaining eye contact with others, keeping in contact with others
Unhealthy anger	Unhealthy	Shouting, bad mouthing another person to others
Healthy anger	Healthy	Assertion, discussing the way in which you have been treated without bad mouthing the other
Unhealthy jealousy	Unhealthy	Prolonged suspicious questioning of the other
Healthy jealousy	Healthy	Brief open-minded questioning of the other
Unhealthy envy	Unhealthy	Spoiling the other's enjoyment of the desired possession
Healthy envy	Healthy	Striving to gain a similar possession for oneself

Table 4.4 Thinking consequences associated with unhealthy and healthy negative emotions.

Emotion	*Thinking consequence*
Anxiety	Overestimates negative features of the threat
Concern	Views the threat realistically
Depression	Only sees pain and blackness in the future
Sadness	Able to look into the future with hope
Guilt	Assumes more personal responsibility than the situation warrants
Remorse	Assumes appropriate level of personal responsibility
Hurt	Thinks that the other has to put things right of their own accord first
Sorrow	Does not think that the other has to make the first move
Shame	Overestimates the 'shamefulness' of what has been revealed
Disappointment	Sees what has been revealed in a compassionate, self-accepting context
Unhealthy anger	Sees malicious intent in the motives of others, whether or not there is evidence of this inference
Healthy anger	Does not see malicious intent in the motives of others, unless there is evidence of this inference
Unhealthy jealousy	Tends to see threats to one's relationship when none really exist
Healthy jealousy	Tends not to see threats to one's relationship unless they really exist
Unhealthy envy	Tends to denigrate the value of the desired possession
Healthy envy	Honestly admits to oneself that one wants the desired possession

most closely related to your chosen type of thinking. Once again if the negative emotion is unhealthy this is, in all probability, your major UNE. If the negative emotion is healthy then again you may have responded constructively in the situation, in which case you may not, in retrospect, have chosen a very good specific example of emotional disturbance.

If you were originally unsure what you felt in the situation under consideration and you have arrived at the same UNE using all three of the above methods, you can be sure that you have selected the right emotion at *C*. If you arrived at the same UNE twice then you probably have selected the right UNE, but if you chose a different emotion every time then I suggest that you choose a different specific example to assess the problem because the one you have chosen isn't providing you with sufficiently clear information.

Those of you who are using this workbook while consulting an REBT therapist will be assisted by your counsellor to identify your major UNE, particularly if you are having difficulty doing so.

Specify how you acted or 'felt like' acting in this situation

After you have identified your major unhealthy negative emotion, you are asked to specify how you acted or 'felt like' acting in the situation under consideration. If you have chosen a specific example of your target problem, then you will have already specified what you did or 'felt like' doing when you formulated your target problem (see Chapter 3). If not, let's consider the two tasks involved here. The first of these tasks is straightforward because it calls upon you to record what you actually did in the situation. The second is a little more complex. It asks you to focus on an inner urge that you did not translate into an overt action. This is known in the professional literature as an action tendency, but most of my clients understand it better when asked to report what they 'felt like' doing even if they didn't actually do it.

In Figure 4.4 write down what you did or felt like doing.

Figure 4.5 shows Oliver's emotional and behavioural consequences. You will recall that Oliver's target problem was

> Whenever I am in the company of authorities, I think that they will criticize me and I become anxious. When this happens I try to find an excuse to withdraw from the situation.

You will see from Figure 4.5 that Oliver's emotional consequence is anxiety, the same as appears in his target problem and his behavioural consequence is 'I feel like running away', again the same as listed in his target problem.

2. **C (Consequences)**: identify your major unhealthy negative emotion in this episode, choose one from: anxiety, depression, shame, guilt, hurt, unhealthy anger, unhealthy jealousy and unhealthy envy. Also specify how you acted (or 'felt like' acting) in this situation

   i) Emotional consequences = *Anxiety.*

   ii) Behavioural consequences = *I 'felt like' running away.*

Figure 4.5 Identifying emotional and behavioural consequences: Oliver's example.

Step 3: identify the critical *A*

So far you have done the following:

1. you have chosen a specific example of your target problem or selected an episode in which you disturbed yourself;
2. you have pinpointed your major unhealthy negative emotion and how you acted or 'felt like' acting in the situation in question (these are known as emotional and behavioural consequences and occur at *C* in the *ABC* framework that we employ in REBT).

Your next step is to identify the aspect of the situation that you were most disturbed about at *C*. In REBT we call this the critical *A*. *A* stands for activating event. In the situation in which you disturbed yourself there are potentially a number of *A*s (or activating events). Only one of them is your critical *A*. If you are using this workbook while consulting an REBT therapist he or she will help you to identify the critical *A* in the specific episode under consideration. Here I will give you some guidelines on how to identify your critical *A* by yourself (see Figure 4.6)

Refer to your target problem

If you are assessing a specific example of your target problem, you may be able to identify your critical *A* by referring back to your target problem. To show you what I mean let's return to Oliver. You may recall that Oliver's target problem was as follows:

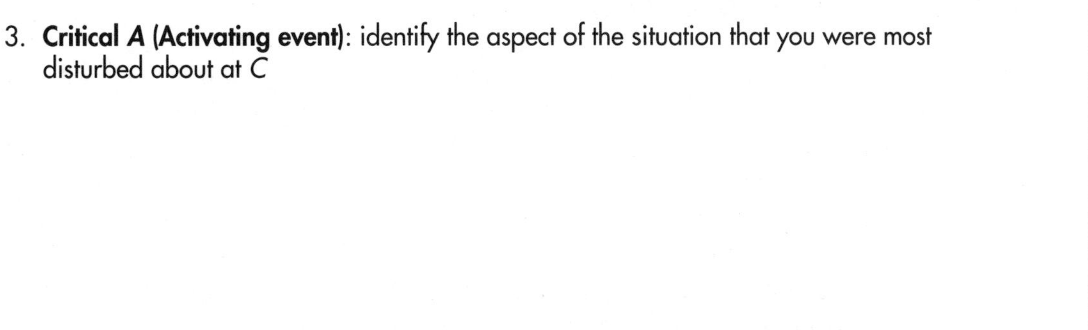
3. **Critical *A* (Activating event)**: identify the aspect of the situation that you were most disturbed about at *C*

Figure 4.6 Identify the critical *A*.

> Whenever I am in the company of authorities, *I think that they will criticize me* and I become anxious. When this happens I try to find an excuse to withdraw from the situation.

The clue to Oliver's critical *A* in the specific example of his target problem is in the theme of this problem, i.e. thinking that authority figures will criticize him. If Oliver has chosen a good specific example of his target problem, it is very likely that the theme of being criticized will be reflected in his assessment of his critical *A* in this example. As can be seen in Figure 4.7 this is the case and Oliver's critical *A* is 'My boss will criticize my work'.

What do you do, however, when your critical *A* is different from the theme expressed in your target problem, or when you are assessing an example of emotional disturbance that is not a specific example of one of the problems on your problem list? In such cases I suggest that you use one of the following three methods.

3. **Critical *A* (Activating event)**: identify the aspect of the situation that you were most disturbed about at *C*

   My boss will criticize my work.

Figure 4.7 Identifying the critical *A*: Oliver's example.

Windy's 'magic' question

My 'magic' question asks you to focus on the situation that you described in step 1 of the DRF-2 and decide what one thing would get rid of, or significantly diminish, the feeling that you listed in step 2 of the DRF-2. In doing so do not say: 'for the situation not to happen', because this will not help to identify your critical *A*. So, assuming that the situation is happening, has happened or will happen, what one thing would get rid of or significantly reduce your unhealthy negative emotion? Once you have answered this 'magic' question, the *opposite* of your answer is, in all probability, your critical *A*.

Let me demonstrate this by referring back to the example of Oliver. You will remember that the situation that Oliver chose to assess was as follows: 'I received a memo to see my boss at the end of the working day'. His major unhealthy negative emotion about this situation was 'anxiety'. If Oliver used the 'magic' question, he would have asked himself

> When I focus on the fact my boss has asked to see me at the end of the day and I feel anxious about this, what one thing would either get rid of my anxiety or significantly reduce it?

His answer would have been 'that my boss will not criticize my work'. The opposite of this answer is 'my boss will criticize my work' which as you can see from Figure 4.7 is Oliver's critical *A*, i.e. what he was most anxious about when he received the memo from his boss.

The listing method

Another approach to identifying your critical *A* is known as the listing method.

1. Focus on the situation that you described in step 1 and on the major unhealthy emotion that you identified in step 2.
2. List all the things that you can think of that you may have been disturbed about in this situation.
3. Review this list and ask yourself 'if I could eliminate or significantly reduce my unhealthy negative emotion by ensuring that one of these items would not occur and by doing so stop my preoccupation with the other items on my list which item would I select?' This selected item would, in all probability, be your critical *A*.

To double check this, reinstate this item to your list and then remove each of the other items one at a time to see the effect of doing so on your feelings. If you think that you would still feel disturbed when the item that you originally removed is the only one that remains then you can be confident that this is your critical *A*.

Let's see how Oliver would have used the listing method. You will once again recall that Oliver's chosen situation was 'I received a memo to see my boss at the end of the working day' and his major unhealthy negative emotion about this situation was 'anxiety'. First, he would list all the things that he may have been anxious about in this situation. Thus, his list may have read as follows:

- my boss will criticize my work;
- he might put me on report;
- he might fire me;
- I might be on the dole for a long time;
- I may never find another job.

Then Oliver would have asked himself the following question:

> If I could eliminate or significantly reduce my anxiety in this situation by ensuring that one of these items would not occur and by doing so stop my preoccupation with the other items on my list which item would I select?

Oliver would have selected 'my boss will criticize my work' as the item that when removed would have eliminated or significantly reduced his anxiety and stopped his preoccupation with the other items on the list. He would then have double checked this by reinstating this item to his list and removing each of the other items one at a time. After each removal he would ask himself whether or not he would still have been anxious and whether or not he would still be anxiously preoccupied with one or more items on the remaining list. If the item 'my boss will criticize my work' remained his chief preoccupation and he was still anxious about this when all the other items had been removed, then his critical *A* was definitely 'my boss will criticize my work' in this situation.

Let me show how Oliver would have double checked his choice of critical *A*.

1 Oliver reinstated his chosen critical *A* and then removed the item 'he might put me on report'

   - my boss will criticize my work;
   - he might fire me;
   - I might be on the dole for a long time;
   - I may never find another job.

   Result still anxious and still preoccupied with the remaining items.

2 Oliver then removed the item 'he might fire me'

- my boss will criticize my work;
- I might be on the dole for a long time;
- I may never find another job.

Result still anxious and still preoccupied with the remaining items.

3 Oliver then removed the item 'I might be on the dole for a long time'

- my boss will criticize my work;
- I may never find another job.

Result still anxious and still preoccupied with the two remaining items.

4 Finally, Oliver removed the item 'I may never find another job'

- my boss will criticize my work.

Result still anxious.

Conclusion Oliver's critical *A* is 'my boss will criticize my work'.

You may be wondering about the status of the other thoughts that Oliver listed. In REBT they are known as thinking consequences of irrational beliefs. Like emotional and behavioural consequences of irrational beliefs, they cease being a problem once you have successfully challenged and changed your irrational beliefs about your chosen critical *A*. Those of you who are using this workbook in conjunction with REBT consultations can discuss the role of these consequences in your psychological problems with your therapist.

Going for broke

The final method of identifying the critical *A* that I will discuss is what I call 'going for broke'. This once again requires you to focus on the situation that you outlined in step 1 and the unhealthy negative emotion that you listed in step 2. Then ask yourself the question 'what was I most anxious (or whatever your emotion was) about in the situation?' The answer, if you are accurate, is your critical *A*.

If Oliver were to have used the going for broke method, he would have focused on the situation where he received a memo to see his boss at the end of the working day and the fact that he was anxious in this situation and asked himself the question 'what was I most anxious about in this situation?' His answer would have been 'my boss will criticize my work' which was his critical *A*.

You may double check the information that you obtained from the 'going for broke' method by using either Windy's magic question or the listing method.

Step 4: identify your irrational beliefs about your critical *A* and their rational alternatives

Identify your irrational beliefs

You have now identified the *A* and the *C* components of the specific example of your target problem (or of any situation that you are assessing in which you felt disturbed). You will remember from Chapter 1 that the REBT view of psychological problems is that *A* (the critical activating event) contributes to *C* (your unhealthy negative emotional and unconstructive behavioural responses) but does not explain the existence of these responses. Rather, these responses are largely determined by your irrational beliefs. I have discussed the nature of these irrational beliefs and their rational alternatives in Chapter 1 and I suggest that you re-read that material if necessary before you proceed.

Step 4 first asks you to identify your irrational beliefs about your critical *A* and to write these down on the left-hand side of this step (see Figure 4.8). As you do so, it is important that your critical *A* appears in each of the irrational beliefs. Here are some guidelines to help you to complete this section.

1 When you complete the demand section bear in mind that a demand is rigid and can take the following forms:

- must
- have to
- got to
- need
- it is absolutely essential that
- absolutely should (it is the word 'absolutely' here that makes the 'should' rigid)
- ought to
- it is an absolute necessity that
- it is absolutely crucial that.

2 When you complete the awfulizing belief section bear in mind that an awfulizing belief is extreme and can take the following forms:

- it is awful that
- it is terrible that

4. ***B* (Beliefs)**: identify your irrational beliefs about *A*

   i) **Demand =**

   ii) **Awfulizing belief =**

   iii) **Low frustration tolerance belief =**

   iv) **Depreciation belief =**

Figure 4.8 Identify your irrational beliefs about *A*.

- it is the end of the world that
- it is horrible that.

3 When you complete the low frustration tolerance (LFT) belief section bear in mind that an LFT belief is also extreme and can take the following forms:

- it is unbearable that
- I can't bear it
- it is intolerable that
- I can't tolerate it
- I can't stand it
- it is unendurable that
- I couldn't endure it.

4 When you complete the depreciation section it is important that you decide whether you are depreciating yourself, another person/other people or life conditions. Also, bear in mind that when you depreciate a person you are making a negative rating of the whole of that person (for example 'I am a bad person') rather than a part of the person (for example 'I am a bad mother'). Finally, depreciating beliefs can also be of the 'less' variety. Thus, both 'I am worthless for failing my exam' and 'I am less worthy for failing my exam' are depreciating beliefs because in both I am giving myself a global negative rating. The content of the rating will also vary and is different with different UNEs. Thus, if your UNE is shame you tend to evaluate yourself as defective, insignificant or disgusting, whereas in guilt you tend to evaluate yourself as bad or rotten. Other person ratings include unlovable, worthless, incompetent, useless, stupid, a fool, no good and pathetic.

Figure 4.9 shows how Oliver completed the left-hand part of step 4.

4. ***B* (Beliefs)**: identify your irrational beliefs about *A*

i) **Demand** =
My boss must not criticize my work.

ii) **Awfulizing belief** =
It would truly be awful if my boss criticized my work.

iii) **Low frustration tolerance belief** =
I couldn't bear it if my boss criticized my work.

iv) **Depreciation belief** =
If my boss criticized my work, it would prove that I was a stupid person.

Figure 4.9 Oliver's irrational beliefs about *A*.

Identify the rational alternatives to your irrational beliefs

Step 4 then calls upon you to identify the rational alternatives to these irrational beliefs and to write these down on the right-hand side of this step (see Figure 4.10). Once again, make sure that your critical *A* appears in each of the rational beliefs. Here are some guidelines to help you to complete this section. I will refer to Oliver's completed right-hand section of Step 4 to exemplify these guidelines (see Figure 4.11).

1 When you complete the full preference section, you need to do two things. First, you need to assert what you want to happen (or don't want to happen) with respect to the critical *A*, for example 'I don't want my boss to criticize my work' which is known as a partial preference. Then you

4. ***B* (Beliefs)**: identify your irrational beliefs about *A* and list their rational alternatives	
i) **Demand =**	i) **Full preference =**
ii) **Awfulizing belief =**	ii) **Anti-awfulizing belief =**
iii) **Low frustration tolerance belief =**	iii) **High frustration tolerance belief =**
iv) **Depreciation belief =**	iv) **Acceptance belief =**

Figure 4.10 Having identified your irrational beliefs about *A*, now list their rational alternatives.

4. ***B* (Beliefs)**: identify your irrational beliefs about *A* and list their rational alternatives

i) **Demand** = *My boss must not criticize my work.*	i) **Full preference** = *I don't want my boss to criticize my work but I'm not immune from such criticism.*
ii) **Awfulizing belief** = *It would truly be awful if my boss criticized my work.*	ii) **Anti-awfulizing belief** = *If my boss criticized my work, it would be bad but certainly not awful.*
iii) **Low frustration tolerance belief** = *I couldn't bear it if my boss criticized my work.*	iii) **High frustration tolerance belief** = *It would be hard for me to bear if my boss criticized my work but I could bear it and it would be worth bearing because it would help me to overcome my oversensitivity to criticism.*
iv) **Depreciation belief** = *If my boss criticized my work, it would prove that I was a stupid person.*	iv) **Acceptance belief** = *If my boss criticized my work, it would not prove that I was a stupid person. It would prove that I was a fallible human being whose work may not have been good enough on that occasion.*

Figure 4.11 Oliver's irrational beliefs and rational beliefs about *A*.

need to negate the demand with respect to the same critical *A*, for example 'but I'm not immune from such criticism'. Your full preference contains both the partial preference and the negation of the demand, i.e. 'I don't want my boss to criticize my work, but I'm not immune from such criticism'.

Bear in mind that a partial preference is flexible and can take the following forms:

- want
- wish
- preference
- desire
- it would be better

- preferably should (the inclusion of the word 'preferably' is important with a flexible 'should').

The above can be positive, for example 'I want', or negative, for example 'I don't want'.

The negation of the demand is also flexible and can take the following forms, all of which you will note begin with the words 'but' or 'however':

- but I don't have to
- but it isn't necessary for you to
- but I'm not immune from
- but you're not exempt from
- however, it isn't absolutely essential that life conditions be that way
- however, it isn't an absolute requirement
- but there's no law which decrees that it must happen
- but it isn't a dire necessity.

2 When you complete the anti-awfulizing belief section you again need to do two things. First, assert that it is bad that the critical *A* has happened (or might happen), for example 'If my boss criticized my work it would be bad'; this is known as a partial anti-awfulizing belief. Then, negate the awfulizing belief, for example 'but hardly truly awful'. Your anti-awfulizing belief contains both the partial anti-awfulizing belief and the negation of the awfulizing belief, for example 'If my boss criticized my work it would be bad, but hardly truly awful'.

Bear in mind that a partial anti-awfulizing belief is non-extreme and can take the following forms:

- it is bad that
- it is unfortunate that
- it would be very unpleasant if
- it would be tragic if.

The above evaluations can vary in intensity from mild to intense.

The negation of the awfulizing belief is also non-extreme and can take the following forms, all of which you will note begin with the words 'but' or 'however':

- but it's not terrible
- but it's not the end of the world
- but it's not awful
- but it's not horrible
- however, it could be worse
- however, good things can come of it.

3 When you complete the high frustration tolerance (HFT) section, this time you need to do three things. First, assert that it is difficult for you to tolerate the critical *A*, for example 'It would be hard for me to bear if my boss criticized my work'; this is known as a partial HFT belief. Second, negate the LFT belief, for example 'but I could bear it'. Third, you need to give reasons why it is worth it to you to tolerate the critical *A*, for example 'and it would be worth bearing because it would help me to overcome my oversensitivity to criticism'. It is worth stressing here that REBT does not advocate that you tolerate anything, rather it encourages you to tolerate only those things that are in your interests to tolerate. Also bear in mind that an HFT belief promotes constructive action and does not encourage resignation when change is possible.

In summary, your HFT belief contains (a) a partial HFT belief, (b) the negation of the LFT belief, and (c) a reason for tolerating the critical *A*, for example 'It would be hard for me to bear if my boss criticized my work, but I could bear it and it would be worth bearing because it would help me to overcome my oversensitivity to criticism'.

Bear in mind that a partial HFT belief is non-extreme and can take the following forms:

- it is a struggle putting up with
- it is hard to bear if
- it is difficult for me to tolerate.

The above evaluations can vary in intensity from mild to intense.

The negation of the LFT belief is also non-extreme and can take the following forms, all of which again begin with the words 'but' or 'however':

- but I can tolerate it
- but I can put up with it
- however, it is bearable
- however, I can endure it.

4 When you complete the acceptance section you need to do two things. First, you need to negate the depreciation belief with respect to the critical *A*, for example 'if my boss criticized my work, it would not prove that I was a stupid person'. Then, you need to assert the acceptance belief 'it would prove that I was a fallible human being whose work may not have been good enough on that occasion'. Your acceptance belief, therefore, contains both a negation of the depreciation belief and an assertion of the acceptance belief: 'if my boss criticized my work, it would not prove that I was a stupid person. It would prove that I was a fallible human being whose work may not have been good enough on that occasion'.

You will recall from Chapter 1 that an acceptance belief acknowledges the complexity, unrateability, uniqueness and fallibility of a human being and the complexity and unrateability of life conditions. Remember this as you formulate your acceptance belief.

To bring this chapter to a close in Figure 4.12 I present Oliver's full *ABC* assessment of his specific example of his target problem.

The Dryden REBT form (DRF-2)

1. **Situation**: briefly describe a specific situation in which you disturbed yourself

   I received a memo to see my boss at the end of the working day.

2. ***C* (Consequences)**: identify your major unhealthy negative emotion in this episode, choose one from : anxiety, depression, shame, guilt, hurt, unhealthy anger, unhealthy jealousy and unhealthy envy. Also specify how you acted (or 'felt like' acting) in this situation

   i) Emotional consequences = *Anxiety.*

   ii) Behavioural consequences = *I 'felt like' running away.*

3. **Critical *A* (Activating event)**: identify the aspect of the situation that you were most disturbed about at *C*

   My boss will criticize my work.

4. ***B* (Beliefs)**: identify your irrational beliefs about *A* and list their rational alternatives

i) **Demand =** *My boss must not criticize my work.*	i) **Full preference =** *I don't want my boss to criticize my work but I'm not immune from such criticism.*
ii) **Awfulizing belief =** *It would truly be awful if my boss criticized my work.*	ii) **Anti-awfulizing belief =** *If my boss criticized my work, it would be bad but certainly not awful.*
iii) **Low frustration tolerance belief =** *I couldn't bear it if my boss criticized my work.*	iii) **High frustration tolerance belief =** *It would be hard for me to bear if my boss criticized my work but I could bear it and it would be worth bearing because it would help me to overcome my oversensitivity to criticism.*
iv) **Depreciation belief =** *If my boss criticized my work, it would prove that I was a stupid person.*	iv) **Acceptance belief =** *If my boss criticized my work, it would not prove that I was a stupid person. It would prove that I was a fallible human being whose work may not have been good enough on that occasion.*

Figure 4.12 Oliver's full *ABC* assessment.

Chapter 5

Setting goals with respect to the specific example

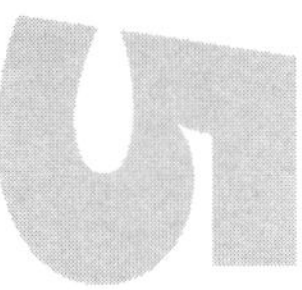

In the previous chapter I taught you how to assess a specific example of one of your target (or other) problems using the *ABC* method. Once you have assessed the specific problem you are working on, the next step is to set goals with respect to this problem. There are a further three steps involved in doing this.

Step 5: select your composite unhealthy and healthy beliefs

In step 4 of the DRF-2 I showed you how to identify the four irrational beliefs that underpinned your emotional and behavioural responses to the critical *A*, and their rational alternatives. In step 5 you are asked to condense these irrational beliefs into a composite, unhealthy belief by selecting the demand and *one* of the following irrational beliefs (awfulizing belief, LFT belief or depreciation belief) that best captured what you believed when you disturbed yourself in the situation in question. There are two reasons why I suggest that your composite unhealthy belief is comprised of these two components. First, if you select just the demand, even though this is at the very core of your disturbance, without one of the other irrational beliefs you will not know whether you are dealing with an example of ego disturbance (where a self-depreciation belief is normally to the fore), an example of other-directed unhealthy anger (where an other-depreciation belief is prominent) or with an example of non-ego disturbance where an awfulizing belief or an LFT belief is normally highlighted in your mind. Second, if you select all four irrational beliefs, you are overloading yourself later when you come to question these beliefs. Questioning a demand and one other irrational belief is manageable, while questioning all four irrational beliefs is usually not. Once you have selected the demand and one other irrational belief, I suggest that you refer to this composite belief as an *unhealthy belief*. From now on, whenever I write about unhealthy beliefs, I refer to beliefs that have a demand and one other irrational belief.

Once you have selected your unhealthy composite belief, go on to identify the rational alternative to this belief. This involves you identifying the full preference and one other rational belief. This latter belief should be the rational alternative to the irrational belief that you selected as the latter part of your composite unhealthy belief. Thus, if this was an awfulizing belief, select the alternative anti-awfulizing belief; if it was an LFT belief select the alternative HFT belief and so on. Once you have selected the full preference and one other rational belief, I suggest that you refer to this composite belief as a *healthy belief*. Again from now on, whenever I write about healthy beliefs, I refer to beliefs that have a full preference and one other rational belief.

I suggest that you use Figure 5.1 to list your composite unhealthy and healthy beliefs. Oliver's composite beliefs are shown in Figure 5.2.

5. **Select your demand** and the one other **irrational belief** (from the remaining three) that was at the core of your emotional and/or behavioural reaction to A. Also **select your full preference** and the **appropriate rational belief** and write down both sets of beliefs (which you can refer to as unhealthy and healthy beliefs respectively) side by side in the space below

Demand and irrational belief *(Unhealthy belief)*	**Full preference and rational belief** *(Healthy belief)*

Figure 5.1 Condense your beliefs.

5. **Select your demand** and the one other **irrational belief** (from the remaining three) that was at the core of your emotional and/or behavioural reaction to A. Also **select your full preference** and the **appropriate rational belief** and write down both sets of beliefs (which you can refer to as unhealthy and healthy beliefs respectively) side by side in the space below

Demand and irrational belief *(Unhealthy Belief)*	**Full preference and rational belief** *(Healthy Belief)*
My boss must not criticize my work and if he does it would prove that I was a stupid person.	*I don't want my boss to criticize my work but I am not immune from such criticism. His criticism would not make me a stupid person. It would prove that I was a fallible human being whose work may not have been good enough on that occasion.*

Figure 5.2 Oliver's unhealthy and healthy beliefs.

Step 6: set your emotional and behavioural goals

The next step is for you to set your emotional and behavioural goals for the specific example under consideration. Ask yourself what would be a healthy emotional and behavioural response to the critical activating event at *A*. Choose responses which are both healthy and realistic and to which you can commit yourself.

In order to do this consult what you wrote in step 2. Select an emotional goal that is the healthy negative emotion (HNE) alternative to the unhealthy negative emotion that you listed in step 2. As before only select one HNE. So, if anxiety was your UNE listed under step 2, select concern as a healthy emotional goal. If it was depression, select sadness and so forth. Table 5.1 lists the eight major unhealthy emotions and their healthy alternatives.

Then choose a healthy behavioural goal, one that is a constructive alternative to the behavioural consequence that you listed in Step 2. Remember that this can either be an overt behaviour or an urge to act, what I refer to in this book as an action tendency. This is not the place to change your critical *A*, you will have a chance to do that later in the book.

List your emotional and behavioural goals in Figure 5.3. Oliver's goals are shown in Figure 5.4. You will note that Oliver considers that feeling concerned (rather than anxious) about the prospect of his boss criticizing his work is a realistic healthy goal and that 'feeling like' attending the meeting is a healthy alternative action tendency to 'feeling like' running away from the meeting.

Table 5.1 Unhealthy negative emotions and their healthy alternatives.

Unhealthy negative emotion	*Healthy negative emotion*
Anxiety	Concern
Depression	Sadness
Shame	Disappointment
Guilt	Remorse
Hurt	Sorrow
Unhealthy anger	Healthy anger
Unhealthy jealousy	Healthy jealousy
Unhealthy envy	Healthy envy

6. **Emotional and behavioural goals**: identify what you would have preferred your healthy negative emotion to have been if you had responded constructively to A. Choose one from concern, sadness, disappointment, remorse, sorrow, healthy anger, healthy jealousy and healthy envy. Also specify how you would have preferred to have acted (or 'felt like' acting) if you had responded constructively to *A*

   i) Emotional goal =

   ii) Behavioural goal =

Figure 5.3 Identify your emotional and behavioural goals.

6. **Emotional and behavioural goals**: identify what you would have preferred your healthy negative emotion to have been if you had responded constructively to A. Choose one from concern, sadness, disappointment, remorse, sorrow, healthy anger, healthy jealousy and healthy envy. Also specify how you would have preferred to have acted (or 'felt like' acting) if you had responded constructively to *A*.

   i) Emotional goal = *Concern*

   ii) Behavioural goal = *I would 'feel like' attending the meeting with my boss to face the music if he wants to criticize my work.*

Figure 5.4 Oliver's emotional and behavioural goals.

Step 7: list your belief goal

The next step is for you to choose the belief (unhealthy or healthy) that you listed in step 5 which you consider will best help you to achieve the emotional and behavioural goals that you outlined in step 6. If you have understood everything so far then you will clearly see that your composite healthy belief will help you to achieve these goals. If you think that your composite unhealthy belief will best help you to achieve these goals then I suggest that you review step 4 of the DRF-2 form discussed in the previous chapter and the material in Chapter 1. Also, discuss this with your REBT therapist if you are consulting one.

When you list your belief goal, do so in Figure 5.5 and make sure that this (healthy) belief is the same as the one that you listed in step 5. Figure 5.6 presents Oliver's belief goal.

Figure 5.7 presents page 2 of the DRF-2 on which you list your goals with respect to the specific example, Figure 5.8 shows Oliver's responses on this form.

You are now in a position to question your unhealthy and healthy beliefs, and this is the topic of Chapter 6.

7. **Belief goal**: which belief listed in step 5 would help you to achieve your emotional and behavioural goals listed above?

Figure 5.5 Identify your belief goal.

7. **Belief goal**: which belief listed in step 5 would help you to achieve your emotional and behavioural goals listed above?

   I don't want my boss to criticize my work, but I am not immune from such criticism. His criticism would not make me a stupid person. It would prove that I was a fallible human being whose work may not have been good enough on that occasion.

Figure 5.6 Oliver's belief goal.

5. **Select your demand** and the one other **irrational belief** (from the remaining three) that was at the core of your emotional and/or behavioural reaction to *A*. Also **select your full preference** and the **appropriate rational belief** and write down both sets of beliefs (which you can refer to as unhealthy and healthy beliefs respectively) side by side in the space below

Demand and irrational belief *(Unhealthy Belief)*	**Full preference and rational belief** *(Healthy Belief)*

6. **Emotional and behavioural goals**: identify what you would have preferred your healthy negative emotion to have been if you had responded constructively to *A*. Choose one from concern, sadness, remorse, disappointment, sorrow, healthy anger, healthy jealousy and healthy envy. Also specify how you would have preferred to have acted (or 'felt like' acting) if you had responded constructively to *A*

   i) Emotional goal =

   ii) Behavioural goal =

7. **Belief goal**: which belief listed in step 5 would help you to achieve your emotional and behavioural goals listed above?

Figure 5.7 Setting goals with respect to the specific example.

5. **Select your demand** and the one other **irrational belief** (from the remaining three) that was at the core of your emotional and/or behavioural reaction to *A*. Also **select your full preference** and the **appropriate rational belief** and write down both sets of beliefs (which you can refer to as unhealthy and healthy beliefs respectively) side by side in the space below

Demand and irrational belief *(Unhealthy Belief)*	**Full preference and rational belief** *(Healthy Belief)*
My boss must not criticize my work and if he does it would prove that I was a stupid person.	*I don't want my boss to criticize my work but I am not immune from such criticism. His criticism would not make me a stupid person. It would prove that I was a fallible human being whose work may not have been good enough on that occasion.*

6. **Emotional and behavioural goals**: identify what you would have preferred your healthy negative emotion to have been if you had responded constructively to *A*. Choose one from concern, sadness, remorse, disappointment, sorrow, healthy anger, healthy jealousy and healthy envy. Also specify how you would have preferred to have acted (or 'felt like' acting) if you had responded constructively to *A*

   i) Emotional goal = *Concern*

   ii) Behavioural goal = *I would 'feel like' attending the meeting with my boss to face the music if he wants to criticize my work.*

7. **Belief goal**: which belief listed in step 5 would help you to achieve your emotional and behavioural goals listed above?

   I don't want my boss to criticize my work but I am not immune from such criticism. His criticism would not make me a stupid person. It would prove that I was a fallible human being whose work may not have been good enough on that occasion.

Figure 5.8 Oliver's goals with respect to his specific example.

Chapter 6

Questioning beliefs

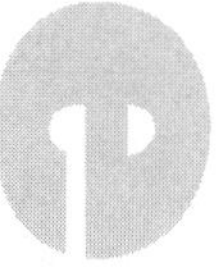

Introduction

Questioning your unhealthy, irrational beliefs and your healthy, rational beliefs is a very important part of REBT. So in this chapter I am going to show you how you can question both your unhealthy beliefs (demands, awfulizing beliefs, low frustration tolerance (LFT) beliefs and depreciation beliefs) and your healthy beliefs (full preferences, anti-awfulizing beliefs, high frustration tolerance (HFT) beliefs and acceptance beliefs). By this point in this workbook, you should (ideally) have grasped what both sets of beliefs are, but if you would like to refresh your memory on this point, let me suggest that you re-read pp. 5–10 in Chapter 1. The purpose of this chapter is to help you to understand why your unhealthy beliefs are unhealthy and why your healthy beliefs are healthy. To do this you need to ask yourself three questions when questioning both sets of beliefs:

1 is it true/false?
2 is it logical/illogical?
3 is it helpful/unhelpful?

What follows will help you to answer these questions.

Please note that it is often helpful to take an unhealthy belief and its healthy alternative and consider them at the same time in the questioning process (this is the approach that I have taken in this workbook). However, you might find it more helpful to question your unhealthy belief separately from your healthy belief. It is worth your while to experiment with both approaches in order to determine which approach is best for you.

Let's now return to the DRF-2. So far you have completed the first seven steps of this form. You are now ready to question your selected irrational belief and rational belief and to do this you need to complete step 8. This is shown in Figure 6.1. Before you do this it is important that you read and re-read the following guidelines for how to question your unhealthy and healthy beliefs. When you have done so, I will provide you with a worked example of how Oliver completed step 8.

Demands versus full preferences

Which are true and which are false?

Demands are false

A demand is rigid and absolutistic while the world is flexible and relative. If a demand were true (e.g. 'I absolutely have to do well in my job'), then there would be no way that I could possibly go against this law (i.e. 'I could not

8. **List persuasive arguments** that would help you to strengthen your conviction in the belief you listed in step 7 above and weaken your conviction in the other belief (see step 5)

   i)

   ii)

   iii)

   iv)

   v)

   vi)

   vii)

   viii)

   ix)

Figure 6.1 Listing persuasive arguments.

possibly fail to do well in my job, even if I wanted to fail'). As there is always a chance that I may go against my demand this proves that the demand only exists in my head and not in reality. It is therefore false.

Full preferences are true

A full preference is flexible and non-absolutistic as is the world. A full preference has two parts:

1 the first part states what I want (e.g. 'I want to do well in my job');
2 the second part negates any demand that I might have (e.g. 'but I don't have to do well').

Now, I can prove that I want to do well, after all this is an inner desire that exists within me. I can also prove that it is desirable for me to do well in my job. Thus, if anyone asks me why it is desirable for me to do well in my job, I can give them reasons to prove that it is desirable (e.g. it increases my chances of promotion and of getting a bonus). Furthermore, I can also prove that I don't have to do well in my job. As discussed above, if there was a law of the universe that states that I have to do well in my job then I would *have* to do well. Not doing well just could not happen. Of course, it is always possible for me not to do well in my job and thus the statement acknowledging this ('but I don't have to do well') is true. So both parts of a full preference are true and therefore the belief is true.

Which are logical and which are illogical?

Demands are illogical

All demands are based on what I call a partial preference. So, in our example, the demand 'I must do well in my job' is based on the partial preference 'I want to do well in my job'. This is a partial preference because it just states what I want. We do not know yet whether the partial preference is really a demand ('and therefore I have to do well) or a full preference ('but I do not have to do well').

Now if we take the two components of a demand – the partial preference component and the demand component – you will see that the latter does not follow logically from the former.

The partial preference component is flexible and the demand component is rigid and it is just not logical for something rigid to follow something flexible. Thus, the statement 'I want to do well in my job' does not lead logically to the statement 'and therefore I have to do well'. So a demand is illogical because it attempts to derive something rigid from something flexible and this cannot be done from a logical point of view.

Thus:

Demand = Partial preference component [flexible] + Demand component [rigid]

for example 'I must do well in my job' (demand) = 'I want to do well in my job' (flexible, partial preference component) + 'and therefore I have to do well' (rigid, demand component).

The demand is illogical because its rigid demand component does not follow logically from its flexible partial preference component:

Flexible → [illogical] → Rigid

for example 'I want to do well in my job' (flexible) → [illogical] → 'and therefore I have to do well' (rigid).

Thus, demands are illogical.

Full preferences are logical

All full preferences are also based on a partial preference. In our example, in the full preference we have (a) the statement 'I want to do well in my job' which is a partial preference and (b) the statement 'but I do not have to do well' which negates the demand.

Now if we take the two components of a full preference: the partial preference component and the negation of the demand component, you will see that the latter does follow logically from the former.

The partial preference component is flexible and the negation of the demand component is also flexible. It is perfectly logical for two flexible components to be linked together. Thus, the statement 'I want to do well in my job' does leads logically to the statement 'but I do not have to do well'. So a full preference is logical because it links together two flexible statements.

Thus:

Full preference = Partial preference component [flexible] + Negation of demand component [flexible]

for example 'I want to do well in my job, but I don't have to do well (full preference) = 'I want to do well in my job' (flexible, partial preference component) + 'but I do not have to do well' (flexible, negation of demand component).

The full preference is logical because its flexible negation of demand component does follow logically from its flexible partial preference component:

Flexible → [logical] → Flexible

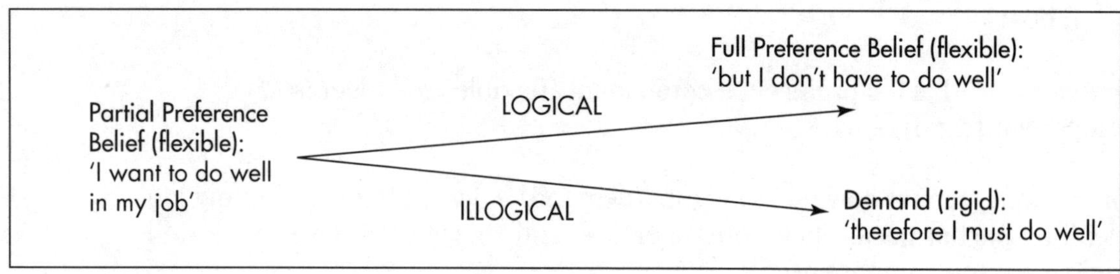

Figure 6.2 Diagram of logical argument – demands versus full preferences.

for example 'I want to do well in my job' (flexible) → [logical] → 'but I don't have to do well' (flexible).

Thus, full preferences are logical.

These arguments are presented in diagrammatic form in Figure 6.2.

Which are helpful and which are unhelpful?

Demands are unhelpful

When you encounter negative activating events demands tend to lead first to one or more of the following *unhealthy* negative emotions: anxiety, depression, guilt, shame, hurt, unhealthy anger, unhealthy jealousy and unhealthy envy, and second, to unconstructive behaviour such as withdrawal, avoidance, overwork, taking no exercise or compulsive exercise, substance abuse and overcompensation. Third, demands tend to lead to subsequent distorted thinking such as overestimating the likelihood of negative events, exaggerating the negativity of events or underestimating your coping resources.

Full preferences are helpful

When you encounter negative activating events full preferences tend to lead first, to one or more of the following *healthy* negative emotions: concern, sadness, remorse, disappointment, sorrow, healthy anger, healthy jealousy and healthy envy, and second, to constructive behaviour such as facing up to and dealing with difficult situations, working sensible hours, and having healthy exercise, eating and drinking patterns. Third, full preferences tend to lead to subsequent realistic thinking such as making realistic estimates of the likelihood of negative events, viewing positive events as equally likely to occur as negative events, seeing negative events in perspective and in a sensible context, and making an objective appraisal of your coping resources.

Awfulizing beliefs versus anti-awfulizing beliefs

Which are true and which are false?

Awfulizing beliefs are false

An awfulizing belief is extreme while the world is non-extreme. If an awfulizing belief were true (e.g. 'It is awful if I don't do well in my job'), then there would be no way that anything could be worse than this because 'awful' in this extreme usage means one or more of the following.

1 100 per cent bad or nothing can be worse. Something can always be worse. As Smokey Robinson's mother used to tell her son: 'From the day you were born 'til you ride in the hearse, there's nothing so bad that it couldn't be worse'.
2 Worse than 100 per cent bad. This is magical nonsense. If we assume for a moment that 100 per cent badness exists, how can anything be worse than 100 per cent bad! The answer is that it can't.
3 It must not be as bad as it is. If it is as bad as it is, then that is the reality. To demand that it must not be as bad as it is goes against reality.
4 No good can possibly come from this situation. No matter how bad something is – like the holocaust – something good can come out of it (for example the determination to learn from this catastrophe and the acts of heroism that it inspired).

When you hold an awfulizing belief you also fail to put things into any kind of perspective. 'It's just awful' and that's that. In doing so you imply that no other perspective matters than the 'awful' one you are now so blinkeredly using. This is obviously false because other perspectives do exist and do matter. Thus, it is possible to put things into a time perspective (e.g. 'Will things appear as bad as they do in 'x' months or years time?') or into a comparative perspective (e.g. 'How does this event compare in badness to other events such as the holocaust?'). When you use these other perspectives you begin to see that what you are evaluating as 'awful' is nothing of the kind.

Anti-awfulizing beliefs are true

An anti-awfulizing belief is non-extreme as is the world, it thus reflects the reality of the way things are. Thus when you are holding an anti-awfulizing belief you think that whatever you are evaluating is one or more of the following.

1 Less than 100 per cent bad. Here you acknowledge that something can always be worse.

2 As bad as it is; no better, no worse. Here you may wish that the situation under consideration weren't as bad as it is, but you aren't demanding that it shouldn't be as bad. Also you realize the following.
3 Good can come from this bad event. Here you appreciate that, in time, some positives may come from this very aversive event and that there are, in all probability, few if any events from which lessons cannot be learned.

When you hold an anti-awfulizing belief you put things into a wider perspective. In doing so, you recognize that when you place the event in a broader time perspective or when you compare it to other aversive events, it is true that the event is bad, but not awful.

Let's look at the proposition that anti-awfulizing beliefs are true in a different way. An anti-awfulizing belief has two parts:

1 the first part states what is bad (e.g. 'It is bad if I don't do well in my job');
2 the second part negates the idea that what is bad is awful (e.g. 'but it is not awful').

Now, I can prove that it is bad if I don't do well, after all I will either not get various things that I want or I will get various things that I don't want. Thus, if anyone asks me why it is bad for me not to do well in my job, I can give him or her reasons to prove that it is bad (e.g. it decreases my chances of promotion and of getting a bonus). Furthermore, I can also prove that it is not awful if I don't do well in my job. As discussed above, if it were true that not doing well in my job was truly awful, nothing could be worse and no good could ever come from this, no matter from which perspective I viewed this event. This is obviously not the case because (a) a minute's reflection will enable me to think of several events that could be worse than not doing well in my job and (b) I could learn from my not doing well in my job and improve my performance.

So when I consider the two parts of my anti-awfulizing belief

1 'It is bad if I don't do well in my job'
2 'but not awful'

I can see that both parts are true and therefore the belief is true.

Which are logical and which are illogical?

Awfulizing beliefs are illogical

All awfulizing beliefs are based on what may be called a partial anti-awfulizing belief. So in our example, the awfulizing belief 'It is awful if I don't do well in my job' is based on the partial anti-awfulizing belief 'It is bad if I don't do well in my job.' This is a partial anti-awfulizing belief because it evaluates the badness of the event in question. We do not know yet whether the partial anti-awfulizing belief is really an awfulizing belief ('and therefore it is awful') or a full anti-awfulizing belief ('but it isn't awful').

Now, if we take the two components of an awfulizing belief – the partial anti-awfulizing component and the awfulizing component – you will see that the latter does not follow logically from the former.

The partial anti-awfulizing component is non-extreme and the awfulizing component is extreme and it is just not logical for something extreme to follow something non-extreme. Thus, the statement 'It is bad if I don't do well in my job' does not lead logically to the statement 'and therefore it is awful'. So an awfulizing belief is illogical because it attempts to derive something extreme from something non-extreme and this cannot be done from a logical point of view.

Thus:

Awfulizing belief = Partial anti-awfulizing component [non-extreme] +
awfulizing component [extreme]

for example 'It is awful if I don't do well in my job' (awfulizing belief) = 'It is bad if I don't do well in my job' (non-extreme, partial anti-awfulizing component) + 'and therefore it is awful' (extreme, awfulizing component).

The awfulizing belief is illogical because its extreme, awfulizing component does not follow logically from its non-extreme, partial anti-awfulizing component:

Non-extreme → [illogical] → Extreme

for example 'It is bad if I don't do well' (non-extreme) → [illogical] → 'and therefore it is awful' (extreme).

Thus awfulizing beliefs are illogical.

Anti-awfulizing beliefs are logical

All anti-awfulizing beliefs are also based on a partial anti-awfulizing belief. In our example, in the full anti-awfulizing belief we have the statement 'It is bad if I don't do well in my job' which is a partial anti-awfulizing belief and the statement 'but it isn't awful' which negates the awfulizing.

Now if we take the two components of an anti-awfulizing belief – the partial anti-awfulizing component and the negation of the awfulizing component – you will see that the latter does follow logically from the former.

The partial anti-awfulizing component is non-extreme and the negation of the awfulizing component is also non-extreme. It is perfectly logical for two non-extreme components to be linked together. Thus, the statement 'It is bad if I don't do well in my job' does lead logically to the statement 'but it isn't awful'. So an anti-awfulizing belief is logical because it links together two non-extreme statements.

Thus:

Anti-awfulizing belief = Partial anti-awfulizing component [non-extreme] + Negation of awfulizing component [non-extreme]

for example 'It is bad if I don't do well in my job, but it isn't awful' (anti-awfulizing belief) = 'It is bad if I don't do well in my job' (non-extreme, partial anti-awfulizing component) + 'but it isn't awful' (non-extreme, negation of awfulizing component).

The anti-awfulizing belief is logical because its non-extreme, negation of awfulizing component does follow logically from its non-extreme, partial anti-awfulizing component:

Non-extreme → [logical] → Non-extreme

for example 'It is bad if I don't do well in my job' (non-extreme) → [logical] → 'but it isn't awful' (non-extreme).

Thus anti-awfulizing beliefs are logical.

These arguments are presented in diagrammatic form in Figure 6.3.

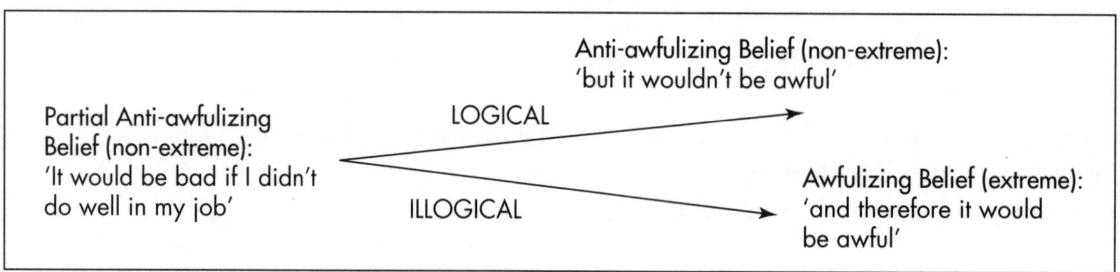

Figure 6.3 Diagram of logical argument – awfulizing beliefs versus anti-awfulizing beliefs.

Which are helpful and which are unhelpful?

Awfulizing beliefs are unhelpful

When you encounter negative activating events awfulizing beliefs tend to lead first, to one or more of the following *unhealthy* negative emotions: anxiety, depression, guilt, shame, hurt, unhealthy anger, unhealthy jealousy and unhealthy envy, and second, to unconstructive behaviour such as withdrawal, avoidance, overwork, taking no exercise or compulsive exercise, substance abuse and overcompensation. Third, awfulizing beliefs tend to lead to subsequent distorted thinking such as overestimating the likelihood of negative events, exaggerating the negativity of events and underestimating your coping resources.

Anti-awfulizing beliefs are helpful

When you encounter negative activating events awfulizing beliefs tend to lead first, to one or more of the following *healthy* negative emotions: concern, sadness, remorse, disappointment, sorrow, healthy anger, healthy jealousy and healthy envy, and second, to constructive behaviour such as facing up to and dealing with difficult situations, working sensible hours and having healthy exercise, eating and drinking patterns. Third, anti-awfulizing beliefs tend to lead to subsequent realistic thinking such as making realistic estimates of the likelihood of negative events, viewing positive events as equally likely to occur as negative events, seeing negative events in perspective and in a sensible context and making an objective appraisal of your coping resources.

Low frustration tolerance beliefs versus high frustration tolerance beliefs

Which are true and which are false?

Low frustration tolerance beliefs are false

A low frustration tolerance (LFT) belief points to our perceived inability to tolerate events. It tends to be false because our ability to tolerate events (particularly if our thinking is healthy) far exceeds this pessimistic perception. If the LFT belief were true (e.g. 'I couldn't stand it if I don't do well in my job'), then there would be no way that I could tolerate this event irrespective of my attitude towards it. Low frustration tolerance in this extreme usage means one or more of the following.

1 Death will ensue. There are very, very few painful events which will actually kill us even if we hold LFT beliefs about them, assuming that we are not in very poor health.
2 Disintegration will occur. This means that we will mentally or physically go to pieces. There is one event which, if encountered, will result in all humans disintegrating. This is sensory deprivation. However, different

people will disintegrate at different speeds. Those holding an LFT belief will disintegrate more quickly than those not holding such a belief. Other than this event, there are probably no events which will inevitably lead to our disintegration irrespective of how we think about them. Ironically, even when you tell yourself that you can't stand something, you are still standing it!

3 Loss of the capacity for happiness will ensue. Even if you encounter trauma, tragedy or catastrophe, it is highly unlikely that you will lose the capacity for happiness. You may think that you will never be happy again but this is evidence that you are holding an LFT belief rather than evidence that you will actually never be happy again. Humans rarely, if ever, lose the capacity to be happy even if they hold LFT beliefs, since this capacity is what helps to define us as human. So, no matter how unhealthily you think, your *capacity* to be happy is not lost. The best way of course to turn this capacity into reality is to develop HFT and other healthy beliefs.

When you hold an LFT belief you adopt a very short-term perspective and fail to consider anything from a longer-term standpoint. However, just because you fail to think of the long term doesn't mean that this long term does not exist. It obviously does and therefore LFT beliefs are false because they do not reflect this reality.

High frustration tolerance beliefs are true

A high frustration tolerance (HFT) belief points to our perceived ability to tolerate events. It tends to be true because our ability to tolerate events is such that we can tolerate and transcend all manner of traumas, tragedies and catastrophes. High frustration tolerance means one or more of the following.

1 Virtually all aversive events (especially highly aversive ones) are difficult to tolerate but they can be tolerated. Therefore you will neither die nor disintegrate if you encounter such events.
2 You may find it difficult to feel happy in the face of aversive events but this does not mean that you have lost the capacity for happiness.

When you hold an HFT belief you are able to adopt a longer-term perspective and can see a future. As such, you are able to consider that whatever it is that you are finding difficult to tolerate is not only tolerable, but is worth tolerating.

Let's look at the proposition that HFT beliefs are true in a different way. An HFT belief has two parts:

1 the first part states what is hard to tolerate (e.g. 'It would be hard to tolerate if I don't do well in my job')
2 the second part negates the idea that what is hard to tolerate is intolerable (e.g. 'but I could tolerate it').

Now, I can prove that not doing well in my job is hard to tolerate, for example, after all I will struggle if I don't do well. Thus, if anyone asks me why not doing well in my job is hard to tolerate, I can give them reasons to prove that it is difficult (e.g. I may have to put in more work to make up for my poor performance, I may have to learn new skills that I don't want to learn or that I may find difficult to learn and I may have my pay reduced so that it would be more of a struggle to make ends meet). Furthermore, I can also prove that failing to do well in my job is not intolerable. As discussed above, if it were true that not doing well in my job was intolerable, I would die or disintegrate or lose my capacity to experience happiness. None of these are likely to be true as a moment's reflection will make clear. Indeed, I can show quite clearly that I won't die, disintegrate or lose my capacity to be happy, for I would gladly face the prospect of not doing well in my job to save the life of any of my loved ones. If it were true that I could not tolerate failing to do well in my job, then I would be far less likely to face this event under these circumstances.

So when I consider the two parts of my HFT belief

1 'It is hard to tolerate not doing well on my job. . . . '
2 ' . . . but I could tolerate it'

I can see that both parts are true and therefore the HFT belief is true.

Which are logical and which are illogical?

Low frustration tolerance beliefs are illogical

All LFT beliefs are based on what may be called a partial HFT belief. So, in our example the LFT belief 'I couldn't stand it if I don't do well in my job' is based on the partial HFT belief 'It is hard to tolerate not doing well in my job. This is a partial HFT belief because it just notes the difficulty of tolerating the aversive event in question. We do not know yet whether the partial HFT belief is really an LFT belief ('and therefore it is intolerable') or a full HFT belief ('but I could tolerate it').

Now if we take the two components of an LFT belief: the partial HFT component and the LFT component, you will see that the latter does not follow logically from the former.

The partial HFT component is non-extreme and the LFT component is extreme and it is just not logical for something extreme to follow something non-extreme. Thus, the statement 'It is difficult for me to tolerate not doing well in my job' does not lead logically to the statement 'and therefore it is intolerable'. So an LFT belief is illogical because it attempts to derive something extreme from something non-extreme and this cannot be done from a logical point of view.

Thus:

LFT belief = Partial HFT component [non-extreme] + LFT component [extreme]

for example 'I couldn't stand it if I don't do well in my job' (LFT belief) = 'It is difficult for me to tolerate not doing well in my job' (non-extreme, partial HFT component) + 'and therefore it is intolerable' (extreme, LFT component).

The LFT belief is illogical because its extreme, LFT component does not follow logically from its non-extreme, partial HFT component:

Non-extreme → [illogical] → Extreme

for example 'It is difficult for me to tolerate not doing well in my job' (non-extreme) → [illogical] → 'and therefore it is intolerable' (extreme).

Thus LFT beliefs are illogical.

High frustration tolerance beliefs are logical

All HFT beliefs are also based on a partial HFT belief. In our example, in the full HFT belief we have the statement 'It is difficult for me to tolerate not doing well in my job' which is a partial HFT belief and the statement 'but I could tolerate it' which negates the LFT.

Now if we take the two components of an HFT belief – the partial HFT component and the negation of the LFT component – you will see that the latter does follow logically from the former.

The partial HFT component is non-extreme and the negation of the LFT component is also non-extreme. It is perfectly logical for two non-extreme components to be linked together. Thus, the statement 'It is difficult for me to tolerate not doing well in my job' does lead logically to the statement 'but I could tolerate it'. So an HFT belief is logical because it links together two non-extreme statements.

Thus:

HFT belief = Partial HFT component [non-extreme] + Negation of LFT component [non-extreme]

for example 'It is difficult for me to tolerate not doing well in my job, but I could tolerate it (HFT belief) = 'It is difficult for me to tolerate not doing well on my job' (non-extreme, partial HFT component) + 'but I could tolerate it' (non-extreme, negation of LFT component).

The HFT belief is logical because its non-extreme, negation of LFT component does follow logically from its non-extreme, partial HFT component:

Non-extreme → [logical] → Non-extreme

for example 'It is difficult for me to tolerate not doing well in my job' (non-extreme) → [logical] → 'but I could tolerate it' (non-extreme).

Thus HFT beliefs are logical.

These arguments are presented in diagrammatic form in Figure 6.4.

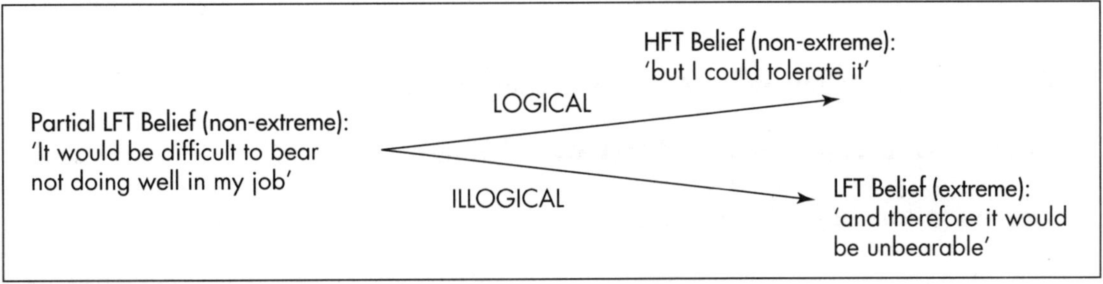

Figure 6.4 Diagram of logical argument – low frustration tolerance beliefs versus high frustration tolerance beliefs.

Which are helpful and which are unhelpful?

Low frustration tolerance beliefs are unhelpful

When you encounter negative activating events LFT beliefs tend to lead first, to one or more of the following *unhealthy* negative emotions: anxiety, depression, guilt, shame, hurt, unhealthy anger, unhealthy jealousy and unhealthy envy, and second, to unconstructive behaviour such as: withdrawal, avoidance, overwork, taking no exercise or compulsive exercise, substance abuse and overcompensation. Third, LFT beliefs tend to lead to subsequent distorted thinking such as overestimating the likelihood of negative events, exaggerating the negativity of events and underestimating your coping resources.

High frustration tolerance beliefs are helpful

When you encounter negative activating events HFT beliefs tend to lead first, to one or more of the following *healthy* negative emotions: concern, sadness, remorse, disappointment, sorrow, healthy anger, healthy jealousy and healthy envy, and second, to constructive behaviour such as: facing up to and dealing with difficult situations, working sensible hours, and having healthy exercise, eating and drinking patterns. Third, HFT beliefs tend to lead to subsequent realistic thinking such as making realistic estimates of the likelihood of negative events, viewing positive events as equally likely to occur as negative events, seeing negative events in perspective and in a sensible context, and making an objective appraisal of your coping resources.

Finally, while there are many things that you can tolerate that are not worth tolerating, HFT beliefs not only stress that you can tolerate the event in question, but also underscore that it is worth it to you to tolerate it. In other words, HFT beliefs encourage you to see that it is in your best interests to tolerate such an event and that doing so will help you to achieve your goals.

Depreciation beliefs versus acceptance beliefs

Which are true and which are false?

Depreciation beliefs are false

A depreciation belief is a static, simplistic global negative evaluation of a complex entity like the self or of a complex set of life circumstances. It is false because it does not take into account the complexity and fluidity of what is being evaluated. In this section I will consider self-depreciation beliefs, although what I say can also be applied to other-depreciation beliefs and depreciation of life conditions beliefs. If a self-depreciation belief were true (e.g. 'Not doing well in my job is bad and proves that I am a failure'), then there would be no way that I could succeed because 'failure' would be my essence or identity. As there is always a chance that I may do well in my job or in other areas, this proves that my self-depreciation belief only exists in my head and not in reality. It is therefore false.

Put another way, self-depreciation beliefs are false because they imply the following.

1 I am a simple organism who can be legitimately given a global rating. This is false because in reality I am a very complex organism.
2 I am a static organism who can be evaluated once and for all. This is false because in reality I am a dynamic organism, changing all the time.

Acceptance beliefs are true

An acceptance belief is an evaluation that reflects the complexity and fluidity of the person or set of life conditions being rated and as such it is true. Once again, in this section I will consider self-acceptance beliefs, although what I say can also be applied to other-acceptance beliefs and acceptance of life conditions beliefs. A self-acceptance belief is true (e.g. 'Not doing well in my job is bad, but does not prove that I am a failure. It proves that I am a unique, fallible human being capable of doing well and not so well'), because it points out that I am fallible, capable of doing well and not doing well. It emphasizes fallibility and uniqueness as my essential features.

A self-acceptance belief has three parts:

1 it evaluates a part of me (e.g. 'Not doing well in my job is bad');
2 it negates that I can be evaluated on the basis of this part (e.g. 'but does not prove that I am a failure');
3 it asserts my essence ('It proves that I am a unique, fallible human being capable of doing well and not so well').

All three parts are true and therefore my self-acceptance belief is true.

Put another way, self-acceptance beliefs are true because they state that:

1 I am a complex organism who cannot be legitimately given a global rating;
2 I am a fluid organism who cannot be evaluated once and for all;
3 my essence is my fallibility and my uniqueness.

Which are logical and which are illogical?

Depreciation beliefs are illogical

Depreciation beliefs comprise two components: a rating of part of your 'self' and a rating of the whole of your 'self'. In the case of a self-depreciation belief, we have:

Self-depreciation belief = Rating of part of 'self' + rating of whole of 'self'

for example 'Not doing well in my job is bad and proves that I am a failure' (self-depreciation belief) = 'Not doing well in my job is bad' (rating of part of 'self') + 'and proves that I am a failure' (rating of whole of 'self').

All depreciation beliefs are illogical because they are based on the part–whole error. When you hold a self-depreciation belief (for example) you imply that it is logical to rate the whole of your 'self' on the basis of a part of your 'self'. Thus, when I say 'Not doing well in my job is bad and proves that I am a failure', I begin by rating a part of my 'self' ('Not doing well in my job is bad') and then use that rating to define the whole of my 'self' ('and proves that I am a failure'). However, rating a part of my 'self' and using that rating to define the whole of my 'self' is illogical because the whole of something may well include other parts. Thus, I cannot logically say that I am a failure (whole) because not doing well in my job is bad (part).

Thus depreciation beliefs are illogical.

Acceptance beliefs are logical

Acceptance beliefs comprise three components:

1 an acceptance of your 'self' component which incorporates
2 a rating of part of your 'self' component and
3 a negation of self-depreciation component.

In the case of a self-acceptance belief we have:

Self-acceptance belief = acceptance of 'self' component — incorporating — rating of part of 'self' component + negation of self-depreciation component

'Not doing well in my job is bad but does not prove that I am a failure. It proves that I am a unique, fallible human being capable of doing well and not so well' (self-acceptance belief) = 'Not doing well in my job is bad' (rating of part of 'self' component) 'but does not prove that I am a failure' (for example negation of self-depreciation component). 'It proves that I am a unique, fallible human being capable of doing well and not so well' (acceptance of 'self' component incorporating rating of part of 'self' component).

All acceptance beliefs are logical because they do not make the part–whole error. When you hold a self-acceptance belief (for example) your rating of part of your 'self' is subsumed in your acceptance of the whole of your 'self'. This is logical because you are saying that the whole includes the part and is not defined by it. Thus, when I say 'Not doing well in my job is bad, but does not prove that I am a failure. It proves that I am a fallible human being capable of doing well and not so well', I begin by rating a part of my 'self' ('Not doing well in my job is bad') and then conclude that my self includes that rating ('and proves that I am a fallible human being capable of doing well and *not so well*') and is not defined by it ('I am not a failure'). My acceptance of my 'self' logically follows from my 'part' rating.

Thus acceptance beliefs are logical.

These arguments are presented in diagrammatic form in Figure 6.5.

Which are helpful and which are unhelpful?

Depreciation beliefs are unhelpful

When you encounter negative activating events self-depreciation beliefs (in this case) tend to lead first, to one or more of the following *unhealthy* negative

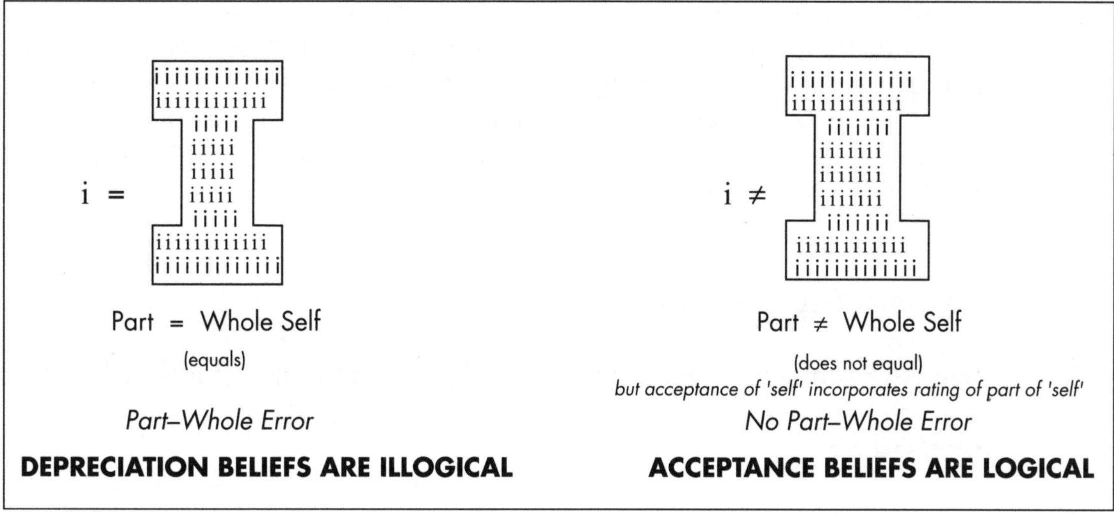

Figure 6.5 Diagram of logical argument – depreciation beliefs versus acceptance beliefs.

emotions: anxiety, depression, guilt, shame, hurt, unhealthy anger, unhealthy jealousy and unhealthy envy, and second, to unconstructive behaviour such as withdrawal, avoidance, overwork, taking no exercise or compulsive exercise, substance abuse and overcompensation. Third, self-depreciation beliefs tend to lead to subsequent distorted thinking such as overestimating the likelihood of negative events, exaggerating the negativity of events and underestimating your coping resources.

Acceptance beliefs are helpful

When you encounter negative activating events self-acceptance beliefs (in this case) tend to lead first, to one or more of the following *healthy* negative emotions: concern, sadness, remorse, disappointment, sorrow, healthy anger, healthy jealousy and healthy envy, and second, to constructive behaviour such as facing up to and dealing with difficult situations, working sensible hours, and having healthy exercise, eating and drinking patterns. Third, self-acceptance beliefs tend to lead to subsequent realistic thinking such as making realistic estimates of the likelihood of negative events, viewing positive events as equally likely to occur as negative events, seeing negative events in perspective and in a sensible context and making an objective appraisal of your coping resources.

You may need to refer to the arguments in this chapter many times before you are able to apply them with ease. I recommend that you devote about 30 minutes a day to self-help and this includes questioning your beliefs until you know in your heart why your healthy beliefs are true, logical and helpful, and why your unhealthy beliefs are false, illogical and unhelpful. After you have done this I suggest that you write down your healthy beliefs on cue cards and review them several times a day and also on occasions when you would otherwise disturb yourself. If you have thoroughly learned the arguments outlined in this text, your use of cue cards will be a meaningful, emotional experience and not a dry, intellectual one.

Worked example of step 8

Figure 6.6 shows how Oliver questioned the unhealthy and healthy beliefs that he selected in step 5. Before I present Figure 6.6 let me remind you what these beliefs were.

Unhealthy belief	**Healthy belief**
My boss must not criticize my work and if he does it would prove that I was a stupid person.	*I don't want my boss to criticize my work, but I am not immune from such criticism. His criticism would not make me a stupid person. It would prove that I was a fallible human being whose work wasn't that good on that occasion.*

Because questioning beliefs is such an important part of REBT let me discuss Oliver's arguments in greater detail.

i) *It would be nice if I were immune from criticism from my boss but I'm not. It is possible for him to criticize me and I'll have to get used to the idea without liking it.*
Comment Here Oliver correctly notes that his full preference is true.

ii) *While I don't want him to criticize me, it doesn't make sense for me to demand that he must not do so. To prefer him not to is flexible, while to demand it is rigid and you can't logically derive something rigid from something flexible.*
Comment Here Oliver correctly notes that his demand is illogical while his full preference is logical.

iii) *As long as I demand that he mustn't criticize me and think I'm stupid if he does, then I'll be anxious about meeting him which won't help me to get on in the company or to focus on doing a good job in my work.*
Comment Here Oliver notes that his unhealthy belief (demand and self-depreciation belief) has dysfunctional consequences for him.

iv) *Wanting my boss, on the other hand, not to criticize me without demanding*

8. **List persuasive arguments** that would help you to strengthen your conviction in the belief you listed in step 7 above and weaken your conviction in the other belief (see step 5)

   i) *It would be nice if I were immune from criticism from my boss, but I'm not. It is possible for him to criticize me and I'll have to get used to the idea without liking it.*

   ii) *While I don't want him to criticize me, it doesn't make sense for me to demand that he must not do so. To prefer him not to is flexible, while to demand it is rigid and you can't logically derive something rigid from something flexible.*

   iii) *As long as I demand that he mustn't criticize me and think I'm stupid if he does, then I'll be anxious about meeting him which won't help me to get on in the company or to focus on doing a good job in my work.*

   iv) *Wanting my boss, on the other hand, not to criticize me without demanding that he mustn't do so will lead me to be healthily concerned and keep me on my toes in a positive way at work.*

   v) *I can prove that I am not a stupid person if my boss criticizes me. His criticism is one act and being stupid would be my essence. One criticism hardly defines my essence.*

   vi) *Conversely, I can prove that I am a fallible human being if my boss criticizes me. I am fallible whether he criticizes me or not. So my identity does not change if he criticizes me. By saying that his criticism makes me a stupid person I am implying that my identity is changed by his criticism.*

   vii) *Even if I acted stupidly at work and my boss is correct to criticize me for my shoddy work, it still does not follow logically that I am a stupid person as a result. For me to conclude this is what philosophers would call a 'part–whole error', the illogical error of defining the whole of something on the basis of a part of it.*

Figure 6.6 Oliver's arguments to strengthen his conviction in his healthy belief.

that he mustn't do so will lead me to be healthily concerned and keep me on my toes in a positive way at work.
Comment Here Oliver notes that his healthy belief (full preference and self-acceptance belief) has functional consequences for him.

v) *I can prove that I am not a stupid person if my boss criticizes me. His criticism is one act and being stupid would be my essence. One criticism hardly defines my essence.*
Comment Here Oliver correctly notes that his self-depreciation belief is false.

vi) *Conversely, I can prove that I am a fallible human being if my boss criticizes me. I am fallible whether he criticizes me or not. So, my identity does not change if he criticizes me. By saying that his criticism makes me a stupid person I am implying that my identity is changed by his criticism.*
Comment Here Oliver correctly notes that his self-acceptance belief is true.

vii) *Even if I acted stupidly at work and my boss is correct to criticize me for my shoddy work, it still does not follow logically that I am a stupid person as a result. For me to conclude this is what philosophers would call a 'part–whole error' – the illogical error of defining the whole of something on the basis of a part of it.*
Comment Here Oliver correctly notes that his self-depreciation belief involves him making the part–whole error which he avoids with his self-acceptance belief.

I want to highlight one important point arising from my comments on Oliver's arguments. Oliver uses the three major arguments that I discussed earlier in this chapter:

1 is it true/false?
2 is it logical/illogical?
3 is it helpful/unhelpful?

and he directs these arguments to the following:

- his unhealthy belief, in this case, demand and self-depreciation belief (see (iii) it is 'unhelpful' argument used)
- his healthy belief, in this case, full preference and self-acceptance belief (see (iv) it is 'helpful' argument used)
- his demand (see (ii) it is 'illogical' argument used)
- his full preference (see (i): it is 'true' argument used)
- his self-depreciation belief (see (v) it is 'false' argument used; see (vii): it is 'illogical' argument used)
- his self-acceptance belief (see (vi) it is 'true' argument used).

Thus, it is possible to create a grid where you can review the arguments that you employed in step 8 of the DRF-2 and plot which argument you employed with which belief. In Table 6.1 I outline a blank grid and in Table 6.2 I plot Oliver's arguments on the grid.

You will note from Oliver's grid in Table 6.2 that he doesn't use all three arguments against all possible beliefs. This is because you don't have to do so. It is important that you use arguments that are persuasive to you rather than all possible arguments. Also, if you use, for example, an 'is it true/false' argument with an unhealthy belief (for example a demand and a self-depreciation belief), you don't have to use the same argument separately with the two components of that unhealthy belief (the demand and the self-depreciation belief). Also some clients like using arguments with the combined belief (healthy and/or unhealthy), whereas other clients prefer to use arguments with the separate belief components. Yet others prefer a mixed approach (which is shown in Oliver's example in Figure 6.6). There is no correct

Table 6.1 Questioning grid

	Is it true/false?	*Is it logical/illogical?*	*Is it helpful/ unhelpful?*
Unhealthy belief (demand + irrational belief)			
Healthy belief (full preference + rational belief)			
Demand			
Full preference			
Awfulizing belief			
Anti-awfulizing belief			
Low frustration tolerance belief			
High frustration tolerance belief			
Self-depreciation belief			
Self-acceptance belief			

Table 6.2 Oliver's questioning grid

	Is it true/false?	*Is it logical/illogical?*	*Is it helpful/ unhelpful?*
Unhealthy belief (demand + irrational belief)	No	No	Yes
Healthy belief (full preference + rational belief)	No	No	Yes
Demand	No	Yes	Yes
Full preference	Yes	No	Yes
Awfulizing belief	N/A	N/A	N/A
Anti-awfulizing belief	N/A	N/A	N/A
Low frustration tolerance belief	N/A	N/A	N/A
High frustration tolerance belief	N/A	N/A	N/A
Self-depreciation belief	Yes	Yes	No
Self-acceptance belief	Yes	No	No

approach so use the approach that makes best sense to you and that allows you to use arguments that you find particularly persuasive.

Once you have digested these points continue your work on your specific target problem by completing Figure 6.1. As you do so don't rely *too* much on the arguments used by Oliver in figure 6.6 Use your own words in constructing your arguments. After you have done this you are ready to move on to Chapter 7.

Chapter 7

Dealing with your doubts, reservations and objections

In the previous chapter you learned how to question your beliefs and, in particular, to generate persuasive arguments to help you to strengthen your conviction in your healthy beliefs and to weaken your conviction in your unhealthy beliefs. Although you may have done this successfully you may still harbour a number of doubts, reservations and objections which may prevent you from moving on. In my experience these doubts, reservations and objections centre on the following:

1 doubts, reservations and objections to adopting your healthy belief and/or giving up your unhealthy belief;
2 doubts, reservations and objections to adopting your healthy negative emotion and/or giving up your unhealthy negative emotion;
3 doubts, reservations and objections to adopting your constructive behavioural goal and/or giving up your unconstructive behaviour.

Unless you identify and deal constructively with any doubts, reservations and objections to adopting your healthy belief, emotion and behaviour and/or giving up your unhealthy belief, emotion and behaviour, then you may stop yourself overcoming your psychological problems. Now I do wish to stress that at this stage in the change process you may not have any doubts about any of the aforementioned points so don't invent any that you don't genuinely have. But if you do have any such doubts, reservations and objections then reading this chapter may help you to identify and deal with them on page 4 of the DRF-2.

What I will do in this chapter is identify the doubts, reservations and objections to adopting healthy beliefs, emotions and behaviours and giving up unhealthy beliefs, emotions and behaviours that clients most frequently express during therapy, and show you how to respond to them. Use what I have written here as an illustration of the kind of doubts that are expressed at this stage of the change process, rather than as a definitive list. If you are consulting an REBT therapist and you don't find your doubt, reservation or objection covered here, then bring up this issue with your therapist.

Finally, don't forget that you are still working at the level of your specific beliefs so that when it comes to identifying your doubts, reservations and objections to adopting your healthy beliefs, emotions and behaviour and to giving up your unhealthy beliefs, emotions and behaviour, you will be asked to specify your doubts, reservations and objections according to the specific belief, emotion or behaviour under consideration .

Having said this, in the absence of knowing your specific doubts I will deal with those that have been most commonly expressed by my clients over the years and this will have to be done at a general level. Consequently you will need to apply my general points to your specific situation.

Dealing with doubts, reservations and objections to adopting your healthy belief and/or giving up your unhealthy belief

In this section I will consider the two major doubts, reservations and objections that people have to adopting each of the four major healthy beliefs and to giving up each of the four alternative unhealthy beliefs that I first discussed in Chapter 1. I will offer responses that you can tailor for your unique situation.

Doubts, reservations and objections to adopting a full preference and to giving up a demand

Doubt 1 My demand motivates me to achieve what I want while the full preference doesn't. Therefore, if I give up my demand in favour of my full preference I'll lose the motivation to do what is important to me.

Response If this were true then I can understand why you would be reluctant to give up your demand and work towards gaining conviction in your full preference. However, your contention is not the case. Let me put it this way. Your demand comprises a partial preference component (e.g. 'I want to do well in my upcoming test') and a demand component ('and therefore I must do so'). Now, the partial preference component provides you with healthy motivation in that it leads you to focus on and execute all the tasks necessary to fulfil your desire (e.g. organizing your study materials, revising these materials and testing yourself to determine your grasp of what you are to be tested on). The demand component, on the other hand, will either provide you with unhealthy motivation, sidetrack you or lead you to freeze.

Let me consider these effects one at a time. First, your demand will provide you with unhealthy motivation. Since you believe that you absolutely have to pass the test you will devote all your energies to studying and neglect other important activities like sleep, rest and recreation that will actually help you to get the most out of your studies. You will likely end up too exhausted to concentrate properly and forget much of what you learned on the day of the test. Second, the demand component will sidetrack you from carrying out effective study and revision strategies and lead you to concentrate on what we psychologists call task-irrelevant thoughts. Thus, you may become overly concerned with the likelihood of failure, exaggerate the consequences of failure and think that the responses of other people to your failure will be highly negative. I hope that you can see that such thoughts are hardly conducive to effective study and test-taking behaviour. Finally, the demand component may lead you to become so preoccupied with failing the test that you may freeze and stop revising for the test altogether.

By contrast, your full preference comprises a partial preference component (e.g. 'I want to do well in my upcoming test') and a negation of the demand component ('but I don't absolutely have to do so'). Now, as before the partial preference component provides you with healthy motivation in that it leads you to focus on and execute all the tasks that you need to do to actualize your desire. The negation of the demand component (a) ensures that you don't get obsessed with passing the test and enables you to take constructive breaks from your preparations; (b) keeps you focused on the task by encouraging task-relevant thinking and (c) prevents freezing.

Doubt 2 My demand indicates what is very important to me, while the alternative full preference fails to do this. Thus, if I give up my demand in favour of my full preference then I will be giving up on what is really important to me.

Response Your demand does indicate what is really important to you, but it mainly indicates that you are rigid and dogmatic about what is important to you. For example, if you hold the following demand 'I absolutely must be treated fairly by my boss' you are indicating two things. You are indeed indicating that being treated fairly by your boss is really important to you. But you are also indicating that his fair treatment of you is absolutely necessary to you and that you absolutely should be exempt from him treating you unfairly. As I showed you in my discussion of the first doubt, it is the partial preference component of your demand that indicates what is important to you (i.e. 'I really want my boss to treat me fairly'). The demand component turns what is important to you into a dogma ('and therefore he absolutely has to treat me fairly').

On the other hand, your full preference indicates in a non-demanding way what is very important to you. Remember that your full preference has two components: a partial preference component ('I really want my boss to treat me fairly') which demonstrates what you consider to be very important to you, and a negation of the demand component which indicates that you have not transformed your strong desire into a dogmatic demand (i.e. 'but sadly this does not mean that he must treat me fairly').

So, giving up your demand in favour of your full preference does not mean that you are giving up on what is very important. All it means is that you recognize that there is no law of the universe that states that you must get what you hold dear.

Also your full preference can be very strong. Thus, I may believe 'I mildly want my boss to treat me well, but he doesn't have to do so' and if I do then I am indicating that my desire is weak. But I am more likely to hold the belief 'I very strongly want my boss to treat me fairly, but that doesn't mean that he has to do so' and when I do I am indicating what is very important to me despite the fact that I am refusing to turn it into a rigid demand. Thus a full preference can and frequently does indicate what you hold very dear to you. This means that you can surrender your demand without losing anything except your rigidity.

Doubts, reservations and objections to adopting an anti-awfulizing belief and to giving up an awfulizing belief

Doubt 1 My awfulizing belief shows that what has happened to me is tragic while the anti-awfulizing belief makes light of this tragedy. Therefore if I surrender my awfulizing belief in favour of the anti-awfulizing alternative, I am making light of what is tragic about my life.

Response This is a commonly expressed doubt but one that is based on a misconception of what constitutes both an awfulizing belief and an anti-awfulizing belief. In order to make my point I am going to make an important distinction between the terms 'tragic' and 'awful' as they are used in REBT. 'Tragic' refers to something that has happened in your life that is highly aversive and which has changed your life for the worse, but has not irrevocably ruined it. Although the event is 'tragic' you can transcend it and go on to live a life with some meaning and happiness. 'Awful', on the other hand, means that something has happened to you that has irrevocably ruined your life which you cannot transcend. As a result your life is devoid of meaning and the possibility of happiness.

Holding an anti-awfulizing belief enables you to acknowledge that you have experienced something that is tragic but not awful according to the above definition. This belief helps you to come to terms with the tragedy and to get on rebuilding your life, whereas holding an awfulizing belief means that you think that your life is over and there is nothing that you can do to rebuild it.

I hope that you can see from this discussion that your anti-awfulizing belief does not make light of any tragedy that way befall you. Indeed, it helps you to acknowledge that a tragedy has happened to you, but gives you hope that you can rebuild your life. While your awfulizing belief shows that what has happened to you is tragic, it turns a tragedy into an end-of-the-world experience which you can never get over. Therefore, if you surrender your awfulizing belief in favour of the anti-awfulizing alternative, you are not making light of what is tragic about your life. You are acknowledging the tragedy and helping yourself to transcend it and to move on with your life.

Doubt 2 My awfulizing belief sensibly protects me from threat, while my anti-awfulizing needlessly exposes me to it.

Response This doubt refers to situations where you experience anxiety. According to REBT theory if you hold an awfulizing belief about something that you perceive to be a threat then you will experience anxiety. You will then tend to act to protect yourself from this threat, usually by avoiding the threat. This unfortunately means that you will not be able to discover whether or not your perception of threat is accurate. Also, by avoiding the 'threat' you will not develop constructive ways of dealing with it, should it turn out to be an accurate threat.

By contrast, if you hold an anti-awfulizing belief about something that you perceive to be a threat then you will experience concern. You will then tend to act to protect yourself only if the threat turns out to be real and you are unable to take constructive action to deal effectively with it. This means that you will not avoid the threat the moment that you perceive the situation to be threatening. Rather, you will stay in the situation to test out your hunch that you are facing a threat.

Thus, your awfulizing belief may protect you from threat but not in a sensible way. In fact, because it influences you to take avoidant action as soon as you perceive a threat, you are likely to continue to perceive threat where none may exist. Also, because you don't learn to take effective action to deal with threat, you are likely to continue to perceive threat in similar situations. In short, your awfulizing belief may protect you from threat in the short term, but it increases the likelihood that you will perceive threat in the longer term.

Also your anti-awfulizing belief does not needlessly expose you to threat. It helps you to remain in the situation long enough to determine whether protective or other action is necessary and if so it helps to determine what constructive action to take.

Doubts, reservations and objections to adopting a high frustration tolerance belief and to giving up a low frustration tolerance belief

Doubt 1 If I adopt my high frustration tolerance (HFT) belief I will learn to put up with aversive situations. My low frustration tolerance (LFT) belief discourages me from putting up with these situations. Therefore, I am reluctant to give up my LFT belief in favour of my HFT belief.

Response It is true that holding an HFT belief enables you to tolerate an aversive situation, but it is important that you understand clearly what 'toleration' means here. It does not mean putting up with an aversive situation without attempting to change it. Rather, it means putting up with it while thinking objectively, clearly and creatively about ways of effectively changing it. In other words, holding an HFT belief helps you to deal with an aversive situation. Now, if it transpires that you cannot change this situation then your

HFT belief will encourage you to put up with it without disturbing yourself about it.

By contrast, holding an LFT belief about an aversive situation means that you find the situation intolerable. Consequently you will tend to withdraw from the situation immediately or take impulsive, unconsidered action to try to change the situation that will, in all probability, make the situation worse. If it transpires that you cannot change the aversive situation, which is likely given your impulsive attempts to change it, then you will put up with it while disturbing yourself about it and/or resort to unhealthy ways of distracting yourself from the situation.

In conclusion, adopting your HFT belief helps you to put up with an aversive situation as a means of changing it, if it can be changed, or as a healthy way of adjusting to it if it can't be changed. Your LFT belief tends to decrease your chances of changing the aversive situation and increases the chances that you will disturb yourself in some way if it continues to exist.

Doubt 2 My LFT belief helps me to avoid emotional pain. My HFT belief will expose me to more emotional pain. Therefore I am reluctant to give up my LFT belief in favour of my HFT belief.

Response You are correct when you state that your LFT belief will help you to avoid emotional pain and that your HFT belief will increase your emotional pain, but (and it is a very big 'but') only in the very short term. In the longer term your LFT belief will increase the chances that your life will become very restricted, dominated by avoidance of difficult situations and ineffective ways of dealing with these situations. LFT beliefs tend to result in procrastination, anxiety and substance abuse, to name but a few psychological problems

By contrast your HFT belief will help you to deal with the situations about which you experience emotional pain with the result that your emotional pain will be lessened and when you experience such pain it will be based on healthy negative emotions. LFT beliefs, on the other hand, lead you to experience unhealthy negative emotions. So, if your goal is to rid yourself of immediate emotional pain, don't change your LFT belief. But if your goal is to live a freer, healthier life then change your LFT belief in favour of your HFT belief.

Doubts, reservations and objections to adopting an acceptance belief and to giving up a depreciation belief

Doubt 1 Accepting myself means that I don't need to change aspects of myself that I am not happy with or that I can't change. Depreciating myself, on the other hand, motivates me to change. Therefore, adopting a self-acceptance belief discourages personal change, while keeping my self-depreciation belief encourages such change.

Response You are confusing the term 'acceptance' with the terms 'resignation' and 'complacency'. Accepting yourself means acknowledging that you are a complex, unique fallible human being with good aspects, bad aspects and neutral aspects. It means that you can and are advised to identify aspects of yourself that you are not happy with and to change them if you can. Indeed, adopting a self-acceptance belief will help you to change these aspects because it will enable you to devote all your energies to understanding the factors involved and what you can do to change them (e.g. 'I tend to procrastinate and this proves that I am a fallible human being with good, bad and neutral aspects. Since procrastination is a negative aspect, let me see why I do it and what I can do to stop doing it'). Resignation, on the other hand, means not trying to change negative aspects of yourself because you are sure that you cannot change them (e.g. 'I tend to procrastinate and there is nothing that I can do to change this'). This is very different to what is meant by self-acceptance. Finally, 'complacency' means having an 'I'm alright Jack' philosophy which discourages self-change because there is no need to change anything about you. Again this is very different from self-acceptance.

Holding a self-depreciation belief actually discourages self-change. Depreciating yourself means treating yourself as if you were a simple being whose totality can be rated rather than as a complex, unique fallible human being who cannot legitimately be given a global rating. It means that when you identify a negative aspect of yourself that you wish to change you depreciate yourself for having this aspect (e.g. 'I tend to procrastinate and this proves that I am an incompetent fool'). Adopting a self-depreciation belief will stop you from changing your negative aspects because, rather than devoting all your energies to working to change them, you focus on your negativity as a person. Thus, instead of focusing on reasons why you tend to procrastinate and figuring out a way of dealing with these factors you dwell on what an incompetent fool you are.

Your self-acceptance belief therefore, has the opposite effect to the one you think it has. It motivates you to change aspects of yourself that you dislike rather than thinking that you don't need to change them or that you can't change them. Your self-depreciation belief also has the opposite effect to the one you think it has. It prevents you from changing negative aspects of yourself rather than motivating you to change them.

Doubt 2 Adopting an other-acceptance belief means that I am condoning that person's bad behaviour. Depreciating that person shows that I am not condoning their behaviour.

Response When you accept another person, you are taking the same stance towards them as you are taking towards yourself when you hold a self-acceptance belief. It means that you are acknowledging that the other person is a complex, unique fallible human being with good aspects, bad aspects and neutral aspects. Thus, you can accept the other person without condoning their behaviour. You can therefore acknowledge that your boss is a fallible human being for treating you unfairly without condoning their unfair treatment of you. This attitude will lead you to take constructive action towards your boss if you think that it is appropriate for you to do so.

When you depreciate another person, it is true that you are not condoning their bad behaviour, but it is also true that you are condemning the person for their bad behaviour. Returning to our example, when you hold an other-depreciation belief you don't condone your boss's unfair treatment of you, but you do regard them as a rotten person for treating you badly. This attitude will stop you from taking constructive action towards your boss and may lead you to take action that is harmful to both you and your boss.

In summary, holding an other-acceptance belief does not mean that you are condoning another person's bad behaviour. It also has the advantage of promoting constructive action with the person who is acting badly. Holding an other-depreciation belief also does not lead to you condoning the bad behaviour of the other person, but may lead you to act in unconstructive ways towards that person.

Dealing with doubts, reservations and objections to adopting your healthy negative emotion and/or giving up your unhealthy negative emotion

In this section of the chapter I will deal with one or two of the most common doubts, reservations or objections that are expressed with respect to adopting each of the eight healthy negative emotions that I discussed in Chapters 3 and 4 and to giving up the alternative unhealthy negative emotion. As before I will list the doubt and then respond to it. My purpose is to illustrate what such doubts may be and how you can respond to them. You will then have an opportunity to identify and deal with your doubts later in the chapter.

Doubts, reservations and objections to feeling concern and to stopping feeling anxious

Doubt 1 Anxiety helps to motivate me to do well while concern doesn't provide me with much motivation. Therefore if I give up feeling anxious in favour of concern I will lose motivation to do things.

Response Anxiety can gear up your system and motivate you but it often does so at a price. Useful motivation comprises arousal that anxiety does provide and reflective thinking which anxiety often impedes. So when you are anxious you are geared up for action but can't think clearly about what constitutes productive action. Thus, when you are anxious you are often rushing around like a headless chicken, motivated and geared up enough to take action, but flooded with many, often competing, thoughts about what action to take.

By contrast when you feel concern you have both the motivation to take action and the presence of mind to think clearly about what constructive action to take. If you feel concern as opposed to anxiety you are motivated to take action, and can take full advantage of that motivation to deal with the threat you are facing in a considered, constructive way. Anxiety may give you the former but it doesn't give you the latter.

Doubt 2 Anxiety keeps me on my guard, while if I am concerned I am lulled into a false sense of security. Therefore I need to feel anxious in order to be alert to threat.

Response It is true that anxiety keeps you on your guard, but it often leads you to overestimate both the presence of the threat and the extent of the threat. Thus, if you tend to feel anxious about what people think of you, when you meet a new group of people you tend to think that many of these people will not like you. You may then focus on evidence in the environment that you think confirms your perception (e.g. you may infer that because a person does not smile at you it is evidence that he or she does not like you) and edit out or distort evidence that is inconsistent with your perception (e.g. you may think that a person being nice to you is evidence that he or she feels sorry for you). One might say that when you are anxious you lull yourself into a false sense of *insecurity*.

By contrast, when you feel concern, rather than anxiety, you are a lot more realistic in your perception of threat. You tend to see threat when it actually exists and not when it does not exist. Thus, if you tend to feel concerned, but not anxious, about what people think of you, when you meet a new group of people you tend to think a person does not like you only when he or she gives you just cause to make that conclusion. Otherwise you think that they are neutral towards you until they get to know you better. You don't necessarily think that everyone will like you until you get evidence to the contrary. This realistic appraisal means that when you are concerned you do not lull yourself into a false sense of security.

Doubts, reservations and objections to feeling sad and to stopping feeling depressed

Doubt 1 Feeling depressed is an appropriate response to a significant loss. Feeling sad minimizes the significance of my loss. So in order for me to do justice to my loss, I need to feel depressed.

Response If you have experienced a significant loss in your life you may well think that depression is an appropriate response to that loss, but fortunately you would be wrong. I say fortunately here because depression is a disorder of mood that leads to withdrawal from life and despair about the future. This is not a healthy response to loss.

Your doubt about sadness being an appropriate response to a significant loss is based on the idea that sadness is of mild or moderate intensity and that such a 'low-level' intensity does not do justice to a 'high-level' or significant loss. However, sadness can be an intense emotion that enables you to digest and adjust to your loss without withdrawal from life or despair about the future. As such, sadness is both an appropriate and a healthy emotional response to your significant loss and one that does full justice to the significance of that loss.

Doubt 2 Feeling depressed is evidence that I am sensitive, whereas feeling sad means that I am less sensitive. Thus my depression enables me to keep my sensitivity.

Response Luckily you are wrong about this. Depression is a response to a loss from your personal domain that is based on unhealthy beliefs about that loss. Sadness is a response to the same loss that is based on healthy beliefs. As I have shown you in previous chapters, unhealthy beliefs are characterized by rigid and extreme thinking. Thus, rather than being a sensitive response to a significant loss, depression is more accurately viewed as an *oversensitive* response to that loss. On the other hand, healthy beliefs are characterized by flexible and non-extreme thinking. This means, in this context, that the strength of your healthy belief will vary according to the significance of your loss. Thus, when you experience a significant loss, the strength of your healthy belief will be great and thus you will react sensitively (rather than insensitively or oversensitively) to your loss. In short then sadness is a better sign of your sensitivity than depression which is a sign of your oversensitivity. Thus you will not lose your sensitivity if you work towards feeling sad rather than depressed.

Doubts, reservations and objections to feeling disappointed and to stopping feeling ashamed

Doubt 1 Because I have done something that has seriously broken an accepted social code it is appropriate for me to feel ashamed about what I have done. Feeling disappointed about my behaviour doesn't do it enough justice.

Response When you feel ashamed about your socially inappropriate behaviour you are holding a self-deprecating belief. You believe that you are an inadequate person for what you have done. According to REBT theory this is neither an appropriate nor a healthy response to your socially inappropriate behaviour because you are rating your entire 'self' on the basis of your behaviour (see Chapter 1 for a discussion of self-depreciating beliefs). Remember also that you can feel intensely disappointed about the way you have behaved without depreciating yourself for your behaviour, and we argue in REBT that this intense, but healthy feeling does do justice to your socially inappropriate behaviour.

Doubt 2 The prospect of feeling ashamed about falling short of my ideal helps me to reach my ideal. The prospect of feeling disappointed about falling short of my ideal doesn't motivate me in the same way. So I need to have the threat of feeling ashamed to help me to maintain my high standards of behaviour.

Response This doubt is based on the idea that the threat of depreciating yourself in a shame-based way is an effective way of motivating yourself to achieve your ideal. The prospect of feeling ashamed does have some motivating properties in this sense, but more often it impedes your effort to reach your ideal. As with anxiety, shame (and the threat of experiencing shame) frequently affects your task-oriented behaviour by hijacking your attention with shame-related thoughts. It is difficult to focus on what you are doing (a crucial feature of high-level task performance) when your mind is flooded with shame-related thoughts.

When you are motivated by the prospect of feeling disappointed rather than ashamed about falling short of your ideal, you are able to concentrate on what you need to do to achieve your ideal (which you will do because it is important for you to achieve your ideal) without the interference of shame-based self-depreciating thoughts hijacking your attention.

You may not have had the experience of being motivated by the prospect of feeling disappointed about failing to achieve your ideal, but this does not mean that it is not a more effective motivator than the threat of feeling shame in the same circumstances. Feelings of disappointment are a more effective motivator, but you need to practise acting on your healthy beliefs to appreciate this point.

Doubts, reservations and objections to feeling remorse and to stopping feeling guilt

Doubt 1 Feeling guilty about wrongdoing helps prevent me from breaking my moral code. Feeling remorse about wrongdoing wouldn't have the same effect on me. Therefore I need to feel guilty to stay on the straight and narrow.

Response When you feel guilty about doing something wrong you think that you are a bad person for breaking your moral code. When you think that you are a bad person you make it more, rather than less, likely that you will do bad things. Why? Because if you are a bad person how can you fail to act badly, now and in the future? You can't. On the other hand, when you feel remorseful, but not guilty about breaking your moral code, you do not think of yourself as a bad person. Rather, you accept yourself as a fallible human being and as such you are capable of doing, bad, good and neutral things. Since this self-acceptance belief acknowledges you are capable of acting morally, you are more likely to act well than you are when you depreciate yourself as a bad person. Thus, remorse is more likely to keep you on the straight and narrow than guilt.

Doubt 2 If I don't feel guilty about my wrongdoing then I might turn into a psychopath. Guilt is evidence that I have a conscience.

Response You seem to think that you have two choices in the moral domain, either feel guilty or be a psychopath. However, there is a third, more constructive option – to feel remorse. Let me illustrate what I mean by referring to the following scenarios.

In each case I want you to imagine that you have broken a generally accepted moral code.

1 I have done something wrong – I am a bad person for doing wrong (guilt);
2 I haven't done anything wrong (psychopathy);
3 I have done something wrong – I am a fallible person who has done wrong (remorse).

In the guilt scenario you demonstrate that you have a conscience by acknowledging that you have done something wrong, but you needlessly disturb yourself by globally rating yourself as a bad person. In the psychopathy scenario you do not acknowledge that you have done anything wrong and thus demonstrate that you have no conscience. In the remorse scenario, as in the guilt scenario, you demonstrate that you have a conscience but, unlike in the guilt scenario, you do not needlessly disturb yourself in that you accept yourself as a complex, fallible human being capable of good and bad (as well as neutral) acts.

Thus, remorse prevents you from turning into a psychopath, but it also prevents you from needlessly disturbing yourself.

Doubts, reservations and objections to feeling sorrow and to stopping feeling hurt

Doubt Feeling hurt when I feel betrayed is perfectly normal, so why should I give it up? I don't understand what feeling sorrowful about being betrayed means.

Response Your doubt touches upon the issue that in the English language we do not have very clear, generally agreed terms that keenly distinguish between unhealthy negative emotions (such as hurt) and healthy negative emotions (such as sorrow). Consequently, the terms that I use (e.g. hurt versus sorrow) may not be meaningful to you. If this is the case you can come up with your own words once you have understood the major differences between (what I call) hurt and sorrow. Let me use a common example to make my point.

Imagine that you have told a friend something in confidence and they have agreed to keep your secret to themselves. You then discover that they have revealed your secret to several other people. You correctly conclude that your friend has betrayed you. Now when you feel hurt about this betrayal:

1 you hold one or more of the following unhealthy beliefs;

- my friend absolutely should not have betrayed me
- it's terrible that they betrayed me
- I can't stand the fact that they betrayed me
- I have been treated in a way that I didn't deserve, poor me!

2 you tend to act in the following ways;

- you withdraw from your friend and (to a lesser extent) from the other people they have told
- you refuse to talk to your friend and (to a lesser extent) the others when they approach you
- if you do talk to your friend, you do so aggressively
- you plan to exact revenge on your friend

3 you tend to think in the following ways;

- people are not trustworthy
- I'll never confide in anyone again
- you think about the betrayal obsessively.

Now when you feel sorrowful about this betrayal:

1 you hold one or more of the following healthy beliefs;

- it is very undesirable for my friend to have betrayed me but I'm not exempt from being treated in this way
- it's very unfortunate that they betrayed me but it isn't the end of the world
- my friend betraying me is difficult to bear but I can bear it and it's worth bearing
- I have been treated in a way that I didn't deserve; this behaviour is poor but I'm not a poor pitiable creature

2 you tend to act in the following ways;

- you are wary about approaching your friend and (to a lesser extent) the other people they have told, but are prepared to do so
- you are prepared to talk to your friend to discover why they did it and to tell them your feelings, and to the others involved when they approach you
- if you do talk to your friend you do so assertively rather than aggressively
- you don't plan to exact revenge on your friend, but you are reluctant to tell her any more secrets until you have repaired your relationship and she has regained your trust

3 you tend to think in the following ways;

- some people are not trustworthy but others are
- I will confide in someone again, I won't tar everyone with the same brush but I will be more circumspect
- you think about the betrayal from time to time but not obsessively.

From the above I hope that you can see that while feeling hurt might be a statistically normal response to being betrayed, it is not a particularly healthy one. Also I hope that you can now understand what constitutes sorrow as a response to betrayal and that it is, from a longer-term perspective, a healthier response.

Doubts, reservations and objections to feeling healthy anger and to stopping feeling unhealthy anger

Doubt 1 If someone crosses me I'd be a wimp if I responded with what you call healthy anger. The other person is a bastard and needs to be taught a very severe lesson. So don't ask me to give up my unhealthy anger.

Response At the heart of your criticism is the idea that a response to the person who has crossed you, based on healthy anger, is bound to be a weak response and would prove that you were a wimp if you made it. Responses based on unhealthy anger tend to be aggressive and show no respect for the other person. They may well 'teach the other person a lesson' but they either provoke an aggressive response back or intimidate the other person so that they are scared of you. On the other hand, responses that are based on healthy anger are strong but respectful. These responses tend to be assertive in nature, provoke a dialogue between you and the other person and elicit a respectful response from the other person.

Healthy anger in the form of assertion is not a weak response, it is strong and it yields better interpersonal results for you. You will therefore not be 'a wimp' if you work towards healthy anger.

Doubt 2 I feel very powerful when I am unhealthily angry. I don't get that same buzz with healthy anger. So, if I give up my unhealthy anger I'll lose that buzz.

Response Yes, when you feel unhealthy anger you may well experience a sense of power and while healthy anger will give you a sense of power it may well not be as intense as with unhealthy anger. So you may well lose the intense buzz that accompanies unhealthy anger if you work towards healthy anger. However, this is a price that is probably worth paying for two reasons. First, as I discussed in my response to the previous doubt, healthy anger yields more productive longer-term results than unhealthy anger and second, the power that you experience with unhealthy anger is uncontrolled rather than controlled as is the case with healthy anger. So the question you need to ask yourself is this. Are you willing to give up the intense but short-lasting buzz that you get with unhealthy anger in exchange for the better results that you get with healthy anger?

Doubts, reservations and objections to feeling healthy jealousy and to stopping feeling unhealthy jealousy

Doubt Unhealthy jealousy motivates me to do things that reassure me that my partner isn't having an affair. If I give it up then I won't know for sure what's happening and I can't bear not knowing.

Response Your unhealthy jealousy stems from the belief that you need reassurance that your partner isn't having an affair. To give up your unhealthy jealousy, you will have to question and change your unhealthy belief that you need to know that your partner isn't involved with anyone else and that not knowing what's happening is unbearable. When you work towards feeling healthy jealousy (which you will experience only when you have clear-cut evidence that your partner is having an affair with someone else), you will still face not knowing for sure what your partner is up to, but you will able to bear this and learn not to seek reassurance, this in turn will enable you to think more objectively about what your partner is doing when he/she is out of contact.

Doubts, reservations and objections to feeling healthy envy and to stopping feeling unhealthy envy

Doubt What you call unhealthy envy motivates me to get the things that others have that I want. If I give up feeling this kind of envy then I won't try to get what I want.

Response Your point that unhealthy envy motivates you to get what you want may be true on occasion, but when you get what you want you soon move on to coveting something else that someone has that you don't have. In other words, you don't get over your problem of unhealthy envy by pursuing what you don't have. In fact, the more you act according to the beliefs that underpin your unhealthy envy, the more you operate according to this unhealthy negative emotion.

Your implication that healthy envy won't motivate you to get what you want is false because in healthy envy you have the desire to get what you want and this desire will motivate you. Also, when you are motivated by healthy envy you are pursuing something that you genuinely want and when you do get it you don't immediately switch your attention to coveting something else. Healthy envy, therefore, is motivating and helps you to pursue things that you genuinely want and won't get tired of as soon as you have obtained them.

Dealing with doubts, reservations and objections to adopting constructive behaviour and/or giving up unconstructive behaviour

In this section I will consider some common doubts, reservations and objections to adopting constructive behavioural responses to negative situations and to giving up unconstructive behavioural responses. In doing so I will consider two broad categories of behaviour that are frequently found in clinical practice in specific form. As before take what I have to say at a general level and apply it to your own specific, unique situation.

Doubts, reservations and objections to taking action to solve problems and to giving up procrastinating

Doubt 1 If I take action to solve the problem that I face, I may make matters worse, so it is better to wait until I am completely sure that the action I take will be successful.

Response The first part of your statement is correct but the second, your conclusion, is flawed. Thus you may make matters worse if you take action to solve your problem. Given this it makes sense that you give due consideration to what you are going to do to tackle your problem. By all means try to be as sure as you can be before taking action. However putting off taking any action at all until you are completely sure that you will be successful will, in all probability, result in you not solving your problem because you keep putting off doing anything until you are completely sure that your solution will work. How can you ever be completely sure that your chosen problem-solving strategy will be successful? That's right, you can't. By all means take time to think about your problem-solving options until you are as sure as you can be in the circumstances that you will be successful, but don't wait for complete certainty that what you decide to do will work because this is a recipe for ongoing procrastination and the continuation of your problem.

Doubt 2 If I have to take action to solve my problem it is important for me to be in the right frame of mind before I act. So it is better for me to wait until I am in such a frame of mind than to act when I don't feel like acting.

Response My response to this objection to taking action is similar to my previous response. If you wait until you are in the right frame of mind before you take action to solve your problem, you may wait a long time and may miss the best time to act. Also, you may often get into a better frame of mind once you have begun to take action. For example, I do 30 minutes exercise six mornings a week before I start work. When I wake up I am rarely in the right frame of mind to get up and start exercising. Indeed, I am in the right frame of mind to stay in bed and have an extra 30 minutes snooze. However, I routinely go against my immediate frame of mind and exercise. I soon find once I have started that I get into it and become in the right frame of mind to exercise. If I wait until I am in the right frame of mind to exercise before beginning, then I wouldn't exercise.

So recognize that waiting to be in the right frame of mind before taking appropriate action to solve your problem is again a recipe for procrastination and the continued existence of that problem.

Doubts, reservations and objections to asserting myself and to giving up staying quiet

Doubt 1 If I assert myself the other person may get angry with me. So it is better for me to stay quiet and avoid such conflict.

Response Even if you develop a high level of competency at assertion, there is always the risk that the other person will get angry with you and there may be conflict between the two of you. Two issues arise here. First, it is important for you to remind yourself of the advantages of asserting yourself with the person concerned. Second, it sounds like you may have an unhealthy belief about being the object of someone's anger and the resultant conflict (e.g. 'things must be cordial between the other person and myself and I can't stand there being conflict between us'). If so, it is important that you change this belief to its healthy alternative. You will then see that you may be overestimating the likelihood that the other person will get angry with you and that any conflict between the two of you will probably be short-lived and may even strengthen the relationship between the two of you. You will then be more likely to assert yourself.

Doubt 2 If I assert myself, then the other person may dislike me so it is better to stay quiet and avoid being disliked.

Response My response to this doubt is similar to my response to the previous doubt. With assertion there is always the risk that the other person will dislike you. But if you are prepared to stay silent because of a fear of being disliked when it is in your healthy interests to assert yourself, you need to overcome your fear of being disliked by doing the following:

1 identify the unhealthy belief that underpins your fear, for example 'I must not be disliked by the other person, if I am it proves that I am less worthwhile';
2 question this belief and change it to its healthy alternative, i.e. 'I'd prefer not to be disliked by the other person, but I'm not immune from his dislike, if he dislikes me I am not less worthwhile, I am a fallible human being whose worth is constant';
3 remind yourself of the positive reasons for asserting yourself with the other person;
4 take the risk and assert yourself while rehearsing your healthy belief.

Dr Leonard Rorer's contribution

As I was writing this chapter an REBT colleague of mine, Dr Leonard Rorer, published a professional paper (Rorer 1999) on a very similar theme to the subject I have been discussing here, i.e. why people do not change their unhealthy beliefs even though they are able to acknowledge that these beliefs are false, illogical and unhelpful, and that their alternative healthy beliefs are true, logical and helpful. Dr Rorer states that one major reason why people do not change their unhealthy beliefs is that they see there are costs involved in both giving up their unhealthy beliefs and adopting their healthy beliefs. To this end he recommends asking yourself two questions:

1 what would it cost you to give up your unhealthy belief?
2 what would it cost you to adopt your healthy belief?

Perceived negative consequences of adopting a healthy belief: a case example

Dr Rorer argues that one reason why someone is reluctant to adopt a healthy belief is because that person sees negative consequences of doing so. He discusses the case of a woman who was sexually abused by her father and held the unhealthy belief 'My father absolutely should not have abused me'. She could see that such a belief was inconsistent with reality (sadly he did abuse her), illogical (her partial preference not to be abused is flexible and does not logically lead to a rigid demand that this absolutely should not have happened) and unhelpful (she was consumed with resentment) and that her alternative healthy belief 'It would have been much better for me if my father had not abused me, but very sadly this does not mean that he absolutely should not have done so' was true, logical and helpful. However, she 'resisted' adopting her healthy belief in favour of her unhealthy belief. Why? Here's the ensuing dialogue between Dr Rorer and the woman:

DR RORER: What would it mean to you to accept your father? Imagine that you did that. What would the cost be?

WOMAN: It would mean that I would have to allow my daughter to be alone with him, and I know that he would do the same thing to her.

DR RORER: Why would it mean that? Why couldn't you say 'I accept that that is how he is, and that that is what he does,' and also say 'given that I know that, I will not allow my daughter to be alone with him'?

WOMAN: That doesn't make sense, does it? I could. I'll think about that.

And that is just what she did. She saw that she could accept her father, give up her demand *and* take steps to protect her daughter. She planned a visit with her father which turned out to be successful and she reported that she was glad that she made the visit.

What this example shows is that you may think there will be consequences of adopting your healthy belief but, as you look at it, it is possible to adopt this belief and take action to avoid or minimize these consequences, thus enabling you to give up your doubt, reservation or objection to adopting your healthy belief. Bear this important point in mind when you come to identify and deal with your own doubts, reservations and objections about adopting your healthy belief.

Holding on to your unhealthy belief to prevent threatening a deeper cherished belief

You do not hold a beliefs in a vacuum. Rather, your beliefs are linked together in a network of beliefs, and changing one unhealthy belief in favour of its healthy alternative has implications for the rest of this network. Dr Rorer has correctly observed that you may be reluctant to adopt a healthy belief in favour of an unhealthy belief if in your view this poses a threat to another cherished, usually deeper, belief. To illustrate this Dr Rorer discusses the case of a man whose wife had been having an affair about which he was very (unhealthily) angry because he was demanding in a dogmatic fashion that she absolutely must not commit adultery. In the course of therapy it emerged that this man resisted giving up this unhealthy belief (which he did view as unhealthy since it led him to plot diabolical schemes of revenge on his wife and her lover) despite the fact that he had an affair some years earlier, because he considered that doing so meant giving up all his religious beliefs. After much discussion and exploration with Dr Rorer, the man realized that giving up this specific unhealthy belief did not mean giving up all of his religious beliefs and at this point he was able to move forward, adopt the healthy alternative to this belief and let go of his unhealthy anger in favour of its healthy equivalent. As Dr Rorer said, no amount of questioning, challenging or disputing his specific unhealthy belief would have had any effect without him first being helped to see that adopting the healthy belief was not, in fact, a threat to his deeper cherished religious beliefs.

So, if you are doubtful of adopting your healthy belief at the expense of its unhealthy alternative, consider that this adoption may pose a threat to other cherished beliefs in your broader belief system. Ask yourself questions such as 'If I adopt this specific healthy belief would this mean me having to give up or violate another belief in my network of beliefs? If so, which belief is being threatened by adopting my specific healthy belief?' Then find a way of changing your specific belief without violating your deeper, cherished belief. If you are consulting an REBT therapist, discuss this with him/her. If not, discuss the situation with someone objective who doesn't have an axe to grind and can help you to stand back and find a way of preserving your cherished belief while adopting your specific healthy belief.

In summary, your doubts, reservations and objections to adopting healthy beliefs, emotions and behaviour and to giving up unhealthy beliefs, emotions and behaviour are likely to reflect the following.

1 Misconceptions about the nature of healthy and unhealthy beliefs, emotions and behaviour. These misconceptions often take the form of thinking that healthy beliefs, emotions and behaviour have some unhealthy features and failing to see that they are largely healthy, and of thinking that unhealthy beliefs, emotions and behaviours have some healthy features and failing to see that they are largely unhealthy.
2 A focus on the positive consequences of unhealthy beliefs, emotions and behaviour and on the negative consequences of healthy beliefs, emotions and behaviours. In doing so people are often mistaken in their judgements of these consequences, and even when they are correct, these consequences frequently only have such an effect in the shorter term. In making these judgements, people often edit out the predominant long-term disadvantages of unhealthy beliefs, emotions and behaviours and the predominant long-term advantages of healthy beliefs, emotions and behaviours.
3 Threats being posed to deeper cherished beliefs by the prospect of adopting target healthy beliefs in favour of their unhealthy equivalents.

Bear in mind these three general points when investigating your doubts, reservations and objections to adopting healthy beliefs, emotions and behaviour, and to giving up unhealthy beliefs, emotions and behaviour. You can do this in Figure 7.1. Figure 7.2 shows how Oliver did this.

9. Deal with your **doubts, reservations and objections**
Doubts about adopting my healthy belief and/or giving up my unhealthy belief:

Doubt, reservation, objection:

Response:

Doubt, reservation, objection:

Response:

Doubt, reservation, objection:

Response:

Doubt, reservation, objection:

Response:

Doubts about adopting my healthy emotion and/or giving up my unhealthy emotion:

Doubt, reservation, objection:

Response:

Doubt, reservation, objection:

Response:

Doubts about adopting my constructive behaviour and/or giving up my unconstructive behaviour:

Doubt, reservation, objection:

Response:

Doubt, reservation, objection:

Response:

Figure 7.1 Deal with your doubts, reservations and objections.

9. Deal with your **doubts, reservations and objections**
Doubts about adopting my healthy belief: *I don't want my boss to criticize my work but I am not immune from such criticism. His criticism would not make me a stupid person. It would prove that I was a fallible human being whose work wasn't that good on this occasion.*

and/or giving up my unhealthy belief: *My boss must not criticize my work and if he does it would prove that I was a stupid person.*

Doubt, reservation, objection: *But surely people who do stupid things are stupid people.*

Response: *No they're not. They are people who have the capacity to do stupid things as well as non-stupid things. Just like me.*

Doubt, reservation, objection: *But If I'm paid to do well at work, then I must do so. If I give up my 'must', I won't be motivated to do well.*

Response: *I'm paid to do the best I can at work. Being human means that I will act stupidly at times. If I do so too many times then I'll be fired. None of which proves that there is a law of nature decreeing that I must do well at work. I'll certainly strive to do so but I'm not a robot. My fallibility can't be programmed out of me. Also my full preference to do well will motivate me without the anxiety that goes with my demand.*

Doubt, reservation, objection: But I'm using being fallible as a cop out, as an argument to excuse my shoddy work.

Response: *No I'm not. If I have done shoddy work and I'm criticized for it I will take responsibility for my behaviour without regarding myself as stupid. Self-acceptance allows me to do both without copping out.*

Doubts about adopting my healthy emotion: *Concern.*

and/or giving up my unhealthy emotion: *Anxiety.*

Doubt, reservation, objection: *Being concerned about being criticized by my boss might lead me to be complacent at work. My anxiety will ensure that I'm not complacent.*

Response: *Having a 'don't care' attitude will lead to complacency but concern won't. Concern is based on my healthy belief which states that I prefer not to be criticized by my boss. This is not being complacent. It will motivate me to do well at work. My anxiety won't lead me to be complacent but it will impair my performance in a way that concern won't.*

Doubts about adopting my constructive behaviour: *'Feeling like' attending the meeting with my boss to face the music if he wants to criticize my work.*

and/or giving up my unconstructive behaviour: *'Feeling like' running away.*

Doubt, reservation, objection: *Running away allows me to avoid the pain of being criticized. If I face the music I'll give myself more pain.*

Response: *Running away only serves to maintain my problem because it doesn't allow me to face the music while practising my healthy belief. It may give me short-term relief but it won't help me to overcome my anxiety about being criticized in the longer term.*

Figure 7.2 Deal with your doubts, reservations and objections: Oliver's example.

Chapter 8

Taking action

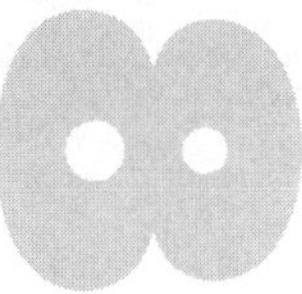

You are now in a position to take what is, in my opinion, one of the most important steps of all in addressing your specific problem, i.e. taking action. The name of the approach to therapy that this book is based on is, as you know, *Rational Emotive Behaviour Therapy.* The word 'rational' points to the fact that thinking is very important in your problems and that thinking rationally is a crucial component in psychological health. The word 'emotive' points to the fact that you are an emotional being and that disturbed feelings have most likely led you to seek help. Finally, the word 'behaviour' points to the fact that change very often doesn't take root unless you act in healthy ways.

Taking action, then, is a very important part of the change process. At this point you have gained some experience in examining your unhealthy beliefs and their healthy alternatives, and you have generated arguments against the former and in support of the latter (as discussed in Chapter 6). You have also had the opportunity to identify and respond to your doubts, reservations and objections to moving forward with your healthy beliefs, emotions and behaviour, and to leaving behind their unhealthy equivalents (as discussed in Chapter 7). The next stage is planning to take action – action that, in particular, is going to strengthen your conviction in your developing healthy beliefs and weaken your conviction in your entrenched unhealthy beliefs. If you are in therapy with an REBT therapist he or she will help you to plan and undertake specific behavioural homework assignments that are designed to help you to act in ways that are consistent with your healthy belief and inconsistent with your unhealthy belief. If you are using this workbook on your own you will still need to take action and the following are some useful pointers to the designing and execution of good behavioural assignments. These guidelines will be useful to you even if you are consulting an REBT therapist.

Guidelines for designing and executing behavioural assignments

Plan to face the critical A

In using the DRF-2 you have been asked to assume temporarily that what was for you the most disturbing aspect of the situation that you were facing was, in fact, true. Thus, in the example that we have been following, on receiving his boss's memo asking to see him at the end of the day (known as the 'situation'), Oliver predicted that his boss planned to criticize his work. This prediction is known as the critical 'activating event' or critical *A* and it is this, rather than the 'situation' itself, that Oliver responded to with anxiety.

In using the DRF-2 form Oliver has assumed temporarily that his critical *A* is true (i.e. that his boss is going to criticize his work) and has proceeded throughout the form on this basis. Oliver continues with this assumption at step 10 of the DRF-2, which asks you to take action on the basis of the work that you have done earlier in steps 1–9. Thus Oliver seeks out his boss assuming that the latter will be critical of his work. If Oliver approached his boss on the assumption that the boss would not criticize his work then he might not be anxious. However in this situation Oliver would not gain practice at feeling concerned, but unanxious about facing his boss's criticism. So, when you are planning to take take action do so while assuming that your critical *A* is true or when it is clear that the situation will definitely include or demonstrate critical *A*.

Avoid safety-seeking strategies

Once you have decided to face the critical *A* do not use any strategies that are designed to seek safety in the situation. For example, once Oliver has decided to face criticism from his boss, then he can act in subtle ways to avoid actually being criticized. Thus he may decide to face his boss at a time when he knows that his boss is likely to be in a good mood and unlikely to criticize him. Or he may begin to criticize his work himself which has the intent of defusing his boss's criticism of this work. In reality Oliver did neither of these things. He deliberately chose to show his boss work that the latter was likely to be critical of at a time when he was most likely to be critical. Now, obviously, Oliver cannot guarantee that his boss will be critical of his work. What he can control is his ability to take steps both to make such criticism likely or unlikely and to seek safety or not. In summary, when you decide to face your critical *A*, take action which increases the chances of that *A* being present in the situation and don't take subtle steps to avoid or minimize the presence of that critical *A*.

Take appropriate risks in facing the critical A

You may be thinking at this point that you don't want to take foolhardy risks in the pursuit of personal change. Thus you may not want to risk losing your job, lose friends or make life difficult for other people. If you are thinking this I fully understand your position and don't want you to take such foolhardy risks. This doesn't mean, however, that you will not be taking some level of risk as you plan to face your critical *A*. Your goal, at this point, is to take an appropriate level of risk. For example, taking the case of Oliver, if he had strong evidence that his boss fires people whose work he is very critical of, then it would represent a foolhardy risk for Oliver to show his boss work that he is likely to criticize at a time when he is likely to be most critical. In such a circumstance, it is likely that Oliver's boss will criticize him in the normal course of events and therefore Oliver does not have to go out of his way to receive critical feedback.

When might you deliberately seek out a negative critical *A* for therapeutic purposes? The following are some suggestions.

1 When the consequences of doing so *may* be negative but not disastrous. In this case you can always practise confronting the critical *A* in your mind's eye without taking unnecessary risks by confronting it in real life.
2 When you have taken steps to avoid confronting the critical *A*.
3 When the critical *A* is unlikely to occur in the normal course of events.

Review your healthy beliefs at appropriate points

Taking constructive action in the face of your target critical *A* is an important step, but the real therapeutic value of doing so occurs when the action is designed to strengthen your conviction in your healthy belief and weaken your conviction in your unhealthy belief. One way of increasing the chance that your chosen action will do this is by reviewing the healthy belief that you are working to adopt. This review process can be done at the following times.

1 *Before facing the critical A.* You can review your healthy belief while you practise facing the critical *A* in your mind's eye and when, for example, you are on your way physically to face the critical *A*. For example, Oliver can say to himself 'I'd prefer my boss not to criticize my work, but he doesn't have to do what I prefer, I can accept myself if he does' while imagining himself talking to his boss and anticipating the boss being critical of his work (see Chapter 11 for a fuller discussion of this technique). He can also write this belief down on a cue card and review it while walking to his boss's office.
2 *During facing the critical A.* While actually facing your critical *A* you can repeat to yourself your healthy belief or a shortened version of it. I recommend the shortened version of your healthy belief when you need to devote much of your attention to, for example, what the other person is saying or the task you are engaged in. Thus Oliver can remind himself that his boss's criticism of his work is evidence that he is fallible while actually facing this criticism.
3 *After facing the critical A.* After facing your critical *A* you can review your healthy belief and consolidate it. Also, if the critical *A* did not occur even though you put yourself into a situation when you thought it would occur, you can still review your healthy belief. For example, if Oliver gave his boss what he considered to be a poor piece of work expecting his boss to criticize this work and his boss was critical of it, after the event Oliver could review his healthy belief as follows 'Yes, my boss did criticize my work and I wished he hadn't, but I'm not immune from his criticism. His criticism does not make me a stupid person. I'm a fallible human being

capable of good and bad work'. However, what could Oliver do if his boss did not criticize this piece of work? He could have told himself the following 'My boss did not criticize my work, but if he had this would have been undesirable, but I am not immune from his criticism. If he had criticized me, it would not have meant that I am a stupid person. It would only prove that I am a fallible human being capable of good and bad work'.

Review your healthy beliefs in different ways

When you come to review your healthy beliefs while taking action, you can do so in two basic ways

1 by varying the audibility of your review
2 by varying the strength of your review.

Varying the audibility of your review

When you vary the audibility of your review you can review your healthy beliefs in three ways:

1 Out loud
2 *sotto voce*
3 silently in your head.

Obviously when other people are around you may not choose to review your healthy beliefs out loud, but when you are alone it is a good idea to do so, particularly in the early stages of personal change. When you are on your own, then, you may wish to begin by stating the healthy belief out loud, proceed to repeating it *sotto voce*, before ending up reviewing it silently in your head. Once you have followed this procedure a number of times reviewing the healthy belief silently in your mind will probably suffice.

Varying the strength of your review

When you review your healthy belief you can do so at various levels of strength.

- Weakly, for example 'If my boss criticizes my work, I am not a stupid person. I am a fallible human being capable of good and bad work'.
- Moderately, for example '*If my boss criticizes my work, I am not a stupid person. I am a fallible human being capable of good and bad work*'.

- Strongly, for example **'If my boss criticizes my work, I am not a stupid person. I am a fallible human being capable of good and bad work'.**

You can review your healthy beliefs at these varying levels of strength out loud, *sotto voce* or silently in your head as shown in the following grid.

A Strongly, out loud	***B*** Strongly, *sotto voce*	***C*** Strongly, silently in your head
D Moderately, out loud	***E*** Moderately, *sotto voce*	***F*** Moderately, silently in your head
G Weakly, out loud	***H*** Weakly, *sotto voce*	***I*** Weakly, silently in your head

The more strongly you review your healthy beliefs, the better (in cases A, B and C). However, as noted above, from a practical point of view it may not always be possible to repeat these beliefs strongly. For example, if you are within earshot of others or you need to devote most of your attention to what you are doing, you may choose to review your healthy beliefs moderately or even weakly. At all other times you will probably find it most persuasive to review your healthy beliefs strongly.

Use imagery to rehearse taking action

Taking constructive action in the face of the critical *A*, while reviewing your healthy beliefs is, as I have said, perhaps the most powerful way of strengthening your conviction in these healthy beliefs and weakening your conviction in their unhealthy alternatives. However, there are two points at which you may wish to use imagery to practise reviewing your healthy beliefs. The first, as I have already shown, involves imagining you are taking action to face your critical *A* while reviewing your healthy beliefs when it is neither possible nor advisable to take action to face the critical *A* in reality (see Chapter 11 for a discussion of rational-emotive imagery).

The second involves using imagery as a way of rehearsing taking action to face *A* in the real world. In such a case I suggest that you take the following steps (I will use Oliver's example to demonstrate this process).

1 Get a clear image of the situation that you are to face and focus particularly on the critical *A* (this, as you will recall, is the aspect of the situation about which you are most disturbed).

Oliver pictures a situation in which he shows his boss a piece of work and focuses on his boss's criticism of this work.

2 Review your healthy belief while focusing on the critical *A* (this could be the full healthy belief or a shortened version).
Oliver focuses on his boss's criticism while telling himself the following.
Full version 'I don't want my boss to criticize my work, but I'm not immune from such criticism. His criticism does not prove that I am a stupid person. It proves that I am a fallible human being whose work may not have been good on this occasion'.
Shortened version 'I can accept myself as fallible in the face of my boss's criticism'.

3 Act in ways that are consistent with your healthy belief and refrain from any behaviour or thoughts that may unwittingly maintain your unhealthy belief.
Oliver sees himself responding to his boss's criticisms by agreeing with valid points and by correcting invalid points in an assertive, polite and non-defensive manner. He sees himself refraining from the temptation of (a) defensively making excuses to justify aspects of his work that his boss was right to criticize, (b) blaming himself in a manner designed to elicit sympathy from his boss and (c) distracting himself from what his boss is saying.

Use role-play to rehearse taking action

If you are consulting a Rational Emotive Behaviour Therapist, you will also be able to practise acting constructively in ways that are consistent with, and therefore strengthening, your conviction in your healthy belief by engaging in role play with your therapist. Here your therapist plays the role of a person who, for example, you are anxious about facing. The therapist's behaviour in this role play embodies the critical *A* in step 3 of the DRF-2. If you are using this workbook alone and are not consulting an REBT therapist, you can still use role play as a rehearsal for later action by asking a sympathetic friend or relative to role play the person whom you intend to face in real life. In doing so, you need to brief your friend or relative in the behaviour that they need to display in the role play. In particular their behaviour needs to embody your critical *A*.

In the following role played scenario with Oliver, I took the role of Oliver's boss and my behaviour was designed to embody Oliver's critical *A*, which as you will recall was 'My boss will criticize my work'. Before we began this role-play I encouraged Oliver to review his healthy belief before we started and at any time during the role play. To this end I advised him to stop the interchange if he thought he was losing sight of his healthy belief so he could give himself time to review out loud, *sotto voce* or silently in his mind. I also told him that I would stop the interchange if I thought that he needed to review his healthy belief.

Before we started I encouraged Oliver to review his healthy belief which he did silently in his mind.

OLIVER You asked to see me?
WINDY (as boss) Yes, I did. I wanted to talk to you about the report that you submitted to me yesterday. I have one or two concerns about it.
OLIVER I'm sorry to hear that.
WINDY (as boss) Now to start with, I thought parts of it were quite sloppy.
OLIVER Can you be more specific? (Previously, Oliver and I had discussed the importance of encouraging his boss to specify his criticisms if he couched them in vague terms.)
WINDY (as boss) Well, let's look at the third paragraph on page 7, it doesn't make sense to me, it really is poorly written.
OLIVER I want to stop the action. I want to review my healthy belief (which he does out loud with moderate strength) *'OK, even if this bit is poorly written, it does not make me a stupid person. My worth isn't dependent on my ability to write well'*. Right that's better, let's resume. Yes, I see you have a point, I can see how I can make that clearer.
WINDY (as boss) Now my real complaint is on the last page. Your conclusion is unclear. I really would have expected someone of your education to write much more clearly.
OLIVER (goes silent)
WINDY (as therapist) You seem at a loss for words.
OLIVER Yes, I'm beginning to put myself down.
WINDY (as therapist) I suggest that you review your healthy belief again, this time perhaps with greater strength. Let me put that criticism to you again, review your healthy belief and then respond. OK?
OLIVER OK.
WINDY (as boss) Now my real complaint is on the last page. Your conclusion is really unclear. I really would have expected someone of your education to write much more clearly.
OLIVER (reviews belief out loud) ***Even if my boss thinks I'm stupid, he's wrong. I'm a fallible human being, damn it, who perhaps could have written the conclusion more clearly.*** Let me have a look at that conclusion. Yes, again, it's not as clear as it could be. . . . Time out again. I really feel the urge to have a go back at him for his dig about 'someone with my education'.
WINDY (as therapist) Resist that urge and concentrate on the conclusion. Review the healthy belief again if you need to.
OLIVER (spends a moment reviewing the healthy belief silently in his mind)

> Well, the conclusion is not a clear as it could be. How about if I have another go at it and show it to you by 11.30 tomorrow morning.

Oliver and I repeated this role play twice more before Oliver felt ready (with some more imagery rehearsal) to risk incurring his boss's criticism in real life by showing him a piece of work which he thought his boss might criticize.

Identify and overcome blocks to taking action

When it comes to taking action which has been designed to strengthen your conviction in your healthy belief, it would be nice if this part of the change process went smoothly. Occasionally it does and you routinely face your critical *A*, take constructive action while doing so and review the appropriate healthy belief. However, it is important to recognize that you may stop yourself from getting the most out of the taking-action phase; when this happens it is important that you acknowledge that this is the case, identify the block and take steps to overcome it. Here are some of the most common blocks to taking action to strengthen your conviction in your healthy belief.

Block 1 'It's too hard'
This is perhaps the most common block to taking constructive action. It is based on a philosophy of low frustration tolerance in which you hold that personal change must either be easy and painless or easier and less painful than it is. Here, you may have done well on following the aforementioned steps on the DRF-2 (although with this philosophy you may have already run into trouble or ground to a halt), but you don't take constructive action because doing so is 'too hard'.

Response An effective response to this block is to do the following:

1 accept the fact, without liking it, that taking action is often difficult and uncomfortable;
2 show yourself that what is difficult and uncomfortable isn't too difficult or too uncomfortable;
3 remind yourself of what you will achieve in the longer term by taking constructive action and what will be the longer term consequences of not doing so;
4 take action.

Block 2 'I might fail'
When you refrain from taking constructive action designed to strengthen your conviction in your healthy belief, you may do so because you fear that your action may lead to failure. Actually, the real block here lies not in the failure

itself but in your attitude towards failure. Here, it is likely that you believe that you must be successful right from the start and if your attempts to take constructive action do not bear positive fruit this proves that you are an inadequate person.

Response An effective response to this block is to do the following:

1 recognise that taking constructive action in the face of *A* is probably new to you and therefore you may well not succeed immediately when you take such action;
2 if you do 'fail', remind yourself that this does not prove that you are inadequate or a failure, but a fallible human being who is able to succeed as well as fail;
3 see your 'failure' as an opportunity to learn more about what you need to do to succeed;
4 utilise this self-accepting philosophy every time that you take action but don't get as much from doing so as you hoped;
5 realise that by following these steps you will increase your chances of strengthening your conviction in your healthy belief, and that not following them will result in you retaining your unhealthy belief.

Dealing with blocks to change often involves you seeking out the unhealthy belief that underpins your resistance, challenging this belief and acting against it. This is exactly the same procedure as when tackling your target problem. Bear this in mind when identifying and dealing with such blocks.

Other blocks The two blocks that I have discussed here represent the most common examples of a low frustration tolerance philosophy, 'It's too hard', and a self-depreciation philosophy, 'I might fail', respectively. Other common blocks are often examples of one or other of these two philosophies as I will briefly show below.

1 *Not facing the critical* A Either by choosing to face a situation in which the critical *A* is unlikely to be present or by focusing on a different, more positive *A* in the situation.
Response Discover whether this subtle avoidance manoeuvre is because of low frustration tolerance or self-depreciation and then respond accordingly.

2 *'I don't feel confident to take action'*
Response Challenge the belief that you need to be confident before taking action and take action unconfidently.

3 *'I'm not sure what will happen if I take action so I'll wait until I know'*

Response Challenge the belief that you have to have certainty before you act and take action uncertainly.

4 *Taking action without reviewing the healthy belief*
Response This may be because of an oversight, in which case review the belief the next time you take action. If not, the block might be a version of 'It's too hard' (e.g. 'It's too hard for me to take action and review the belief at the same time'). This may be realistic and if so, you may need to find short-hand versions of reviewing your healthy belief, for example by consulting a very short version on a 5 × 3 cue card or by keeping one key word in mind (for example 'fallible') which represents the full belief. However, if it is an example of low frustration tolerance respond accordingly.

5 *Taking action and changing* A, *but not reviewing the healthy belief*
Sometimes you may think that you are reviewing your healthy belief while taking constructive action in the face of the critical *A*, but in fact you are not. You are in fact changing A. Let me illustrate what I mean here by returning to Oliver's example.

Let's suppose that Oliver resolved to face up to his boss's criticism and to review his healthy belief while doing so. He hands his boss some work and the boss makes some critical remarks. Now, instead of Oliver reminding himself that he is not immune from his boss's criticism and that he is not stupid in the face of it, imagine that Oliver told himself 'My boss is trying to be constructive. He wants me to do well'. In doing so Oliver has stopped focusing on his boss's criticism as the critical *A* and made a different inference about what his boss actually said (in effect he is not being critical, he is trying to be constructive). This is what we call changing *A* in REBT. In doing so you will note that Oliver does not practise reviewing his healthy belief about being criticized. There is a place in REBT for changing *A* by questioning whether your inference at *A* is the most realistic in the circumstances (in fact, I devote the next chapter to this topic). However, this is usually (although not always) reserved until you have had an extended opportunity to practise reviewing your healthy belief in the face of the critical *A* about which you originally disturbed yourself.
Response Make sure that you keep assuming (temporarily) that your critical *A* is correct and review your healthy belief while taking constructive action. You may find that referring to a cue card on which you have written your healthy belief helps you to keep focused on this belief.

Let me stress again that the blocks I have discussed here are illustrative rather than exhaustive. If you are consulting an REBT therapist and don't find your block covered here, discuss it with your therapist. If you are using this workbook on your own and your particular block hasn't been addressed here, then I suggest you do the following. Imagine that a good friend has told you about the same block to taking actions and has asked you for advice about how to overcome it. Write down what you would say to him or her and then follow your own good advice! You can use this simple technique, of course, even if you are consulting an REBT therapist.

The importance of repetition

It would be nice, wouldn't it, if you could change your unhealthy belief to its healthy equivalent by taking constructive action and reviewing the healthy belief once. Sadly, personal change is rarely so easy and the gains that you make as you embark on a programme of personal change, whether on your own or with a therapist, are usually hard won. Think about the matter as follows. Consider how often over the years you have practised the unhealthy belief that you have targeted to change, both in thought and in deed. When I put it like this to Oliver, he realized that he had held his unhealthy belief about being criticized by his boss (and other authority figures) for many years and he had often reinforced this belief by a number of unconstructive behaviours designed to protect himself from criticism or to disarm his critic if he couldn't avoid criticism. He realized that the effect of such behaviours was to strengthen his unhealthy belief. Thus, it was highly unrealistic for him to expect that he could change his unhealthy belief quickly.

If you want to change your unhealthy belief and strengthen your conviction in the alternative healthy belief, it is important to follow the repetition principle. This simply means that you undertake to practise repeatedly acting constructively in the face of *A*, while reviewing your healthy belief at appropriate points. Thus, Oliver would undertake to show his work to his boss, and to other people who might criticize it, and he would do so a number of times until he gains conviction in his healthy belief. In doing so, he would of course need to show good sense for it would not be wise for him to be sacked from his job because he only showed poor work to his boss. So, it is important to temper repeated practice with a realistic appraisal of its likely consequences. In making a judgement on this issue it is helpful once again to imagine that you are advising a friend who has asked you for an opinion on what constitutes sensible versus foolhardy risk taking on this point.

Where the risks of such repeated practice are low then steady repeated practice along the lines discussed above is recommended. When such risks are realistically high you are advised to gain repeated practice while imagining you are facing your critical *A*, rather than facing it in reality.

Capitalize on change by branching out into related areas

Once you have made progress in strengthening your conviction in your healthy belief about your specific critical *A*, you can capitalize on this by taking action in relevant areas that reflect the theme of your critical *A*. Let me explain what I mean by referring again to the case of Oliver.

Capitalize on your gains I: same theme, similar context, different people

One way of capitalizing on your gains is to extend your practice into similar contexts where different people are involved. Oliver, you will recall, practised facing his boss's criticism at work and acting constructively in the face of it. Here the ingredients can be detailed as follows:

- *theme of critical* A criticism of work
- *context* work
- *person/people* boss.

Now, if Oliver has problems with his work being criticized by other people at work, he can extend his gains by reviewing his healthy belief and acting constructively in the face of such criticism. Here he is facing the same critical *A* theme (criticism of work), in a similar context (work), but with different people (work colleagues).

Note that Oliver can do this in reality or in his imagination. As an example of the former, he can show his work colleagues samples of his work while reviewing his healthy belief about his work being criticized, defending himself in the face of unwarranted criticism and by refraining from making excuses for the quality of his work in order to elicit their sympathy. The ingredients here are as follows:

- *theme of critical* A criticism of work
- *context* work
- *person/people* work colleagues.

Capitalize on your gains II: variation on theme, similar context, different people

If Oliver was anxious about being criticized about his appearance at work by his colleagues, he could review a slightly modified version of his healthy belief (modified to take into account the variation in the criticism theme) while asking them for their opinion about the way that he looked and extend his gains in this way (e.g. 'I am not inadequate if some people don't like the way that I look. I am the same fallible person whether they like my appearance or not). Here the ingredients are:

- *theme of critical* A criticism of appearance
- *context* work
- *person/people* work colleagues.

Capitalize on your gains III: variation on theme, different context, different people

Similarly, if Oliver had a problem about being criticized in non-work settings, he could again review a modified version of his healthy belief (to reflect another variation on the criticism theme) and act accordingly. Thus, if he was anxious about being criticized about his social behaviour at a party by people he had just met, he would review his modified healthy belief (e.g. 'I can accept myself even if they criticize me about my behaviour, I don't have to have to have their approval') while speaking up rather than remaining silent and thus not taking a risk. The ingredients are:

- *theme of critical* A criticism of social behaviour
- *context* party
- *person/people* people just met.

I hope that you can see how *you* can extend your gains at thinking healthily in the face of your problem theme across contexts and with different people. Use Figure 8.1 to plan behavioural homework assignments to strengthen your conviction in your healthy belief in the context you identified earlier on the DRF-2, and then in other contexts and with different people in order to extend your gains. Figure 8.2 shows Oliver's planned homework assignments.

10. List **homework assignments** that you can do to strengthen your conviction in your healthy belief and weaken your conviction in your unhealthy belief. Be specific concerning what you will do for homework, when you will do it and where you will do it. The best homework assignments enable you to rehearse your healthy belief while acting in ways that are consistent with it

    i)

    ii)

    iii)

    iv)

    v)

Figure 8.1 Homework assignments.

10. List **homework assignments** that you can do to strengthen your conviction in your healthy belief and weaken your conviction in your unhealthy belief. Be specific concerning what you will do for homework, when you will do it and where you will do it. The best homework assignments enable you to rehearse your healthy belief while acting in ways which are consistent with it

    i) *To start with I'll ask my boss for feedback on work that I think I've done well. I'll do this on Wednesday and Friday at 4 pm after his tea break. In doing so I'll rehearse the belief that I'm not shoddy even if my work is. Rather, I'm a fallible human being who can work more effectively as well as ineffectively.*

    ii) *Then if that goes well I'll do the same with work that I'm not so confident about the week after, also at the same time while rehearsing the same healthy belief.*

    iii) *Then I'll discuss some work ideas that I'm not too confident about with some work colleagues during our morning coffee break. Before and during this I'll show myself that I can accept myself as a fallible human being capable of good and bad work even if they think I'm stupid for coming up with poor work ideas.*

    iv) *If all that goes to plan, I'll extend my learning to the social area. I'll express myself with people that I've just met at a party and practise accepting myself if they criticize my social behaviour. I'll also show myself that while it is nice to be approved, I don't need these people's approval.*

Figure 8.2 Oliver's homework assignments.

Chapter 9

Reconsidering the critical *A*

Up to now, I have encouraged you to assume temporarily that your critical *A* (i.e. the aspect of the situation that you were most disturbed about in the situation under consideration) is true. I have urged you to do this because this is the best way for you to identify the unhealthy irrational beliefs that we in REBT lie believe at the core of your disturbed reactions at *C* in the *ABC* framework. If you were to reconsider your critical *A* earlier in the emotional episode under consideration, you may realize that your interpretation or inference of the situation you were in was distorted and while you may feel better as a result, you would not have gained practice at identifying, challenging and changing your irrational beliefs. Consequently, these beliefs would remain intact and would be triggered the next time you encountered a similar critical *A*.

In addition, because your disturbed feelings stem largely from your unhealthy belief about the critical *A*, rather from *A* itself, your attempts to reconsider the critical *A* while you hold an unhealthy belief about it will be coloured by this belief and any reconsideration of the distorted inference you may have made in the critical *A* will probably be short-ived. Alternatively, once you have made progress at changing your unhealthy belief about the critical *A*, you are likely to be in a more objective frame of mind and it is this frame of mind that best facilitates accurate reconsideration of the critical *A*.

Let me summarize what I have said in diagrammatic form (see Figures 9.1 and 9.2).

Now that you have gained some practice at challenging your unhealthy belief and some practice at acting in ways that are consistent with your healthy belief, you are more likely to be in an objective frame of mind to reconsider the critical *A*, than you would be without gaining such practice. So how do you go

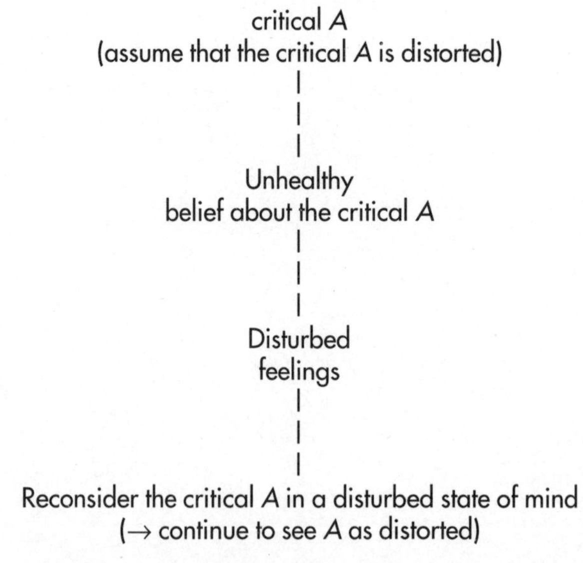

Figure 9.1 Reconsidering the critical *A* without first questioning the unhealthy belief.

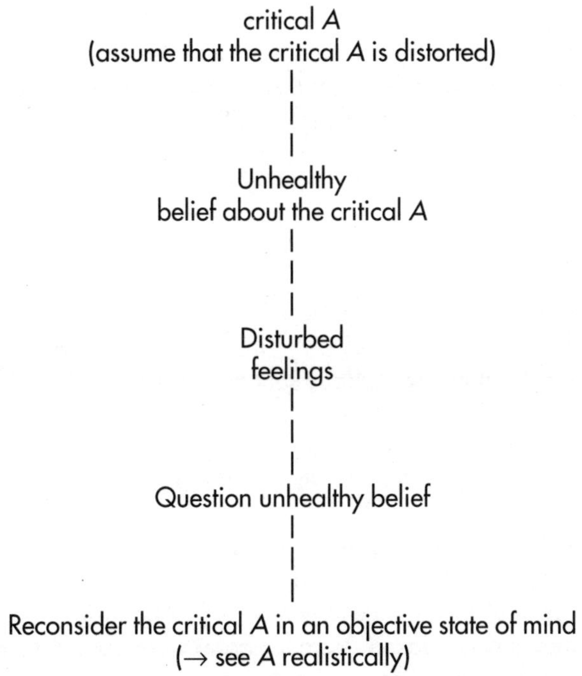

Figure 9.2 Reconsidering the critical *A* after questioning unhealthy belief.

about reconsidering the critical *A*? You do this by going back to it and asking yourself whether or not this was the most realistic way of looking at the situation. This does not mean that we can know for certain that the critical *A* is true or false, for there is rarely any absolute and agreed correct way of viewing an event. What it does mean is that we can weigh up all the evidence that is available to us about the situation at hand and make what is likely to be the 'best bet' about what happened.

There are a number of ways of asking yourself questions to help you reconsider the critical *A* and determine whether or not it was the most realistic way of viewing (i.e. the best bet) what happened in the situation in which you disturbed yourself. I will outline these ways and illustrate them with the case of Oliver (see Figure 9.3).

Write down the situation that you listed in step 1 of the DRF-2 and ask yourself whether what you listed in step 3 of the form was the most realistic way of viewing the situation given all the evidence to hand. This involves considering the inference that you made that forms the critical *A*, considering alternative inferences, evaluating all the possibilities and choosing the most realistic inference.

1 Oliver asked himself how likely it was that receiving a memo from his boss meant that his boss was going to criticize his work. In answering this question he considered the following points.

11. **Reconsider the critical *A***: write down the situation that you listed in step 1 and the critical *A* listed in step 3. Then ask yourself whether or not the critical *A* is the best way of viewing the situation given all the evidence to hand (illustrative questions provided)

Situation: *I received a memo to see my boss at the end of the working day.*

Critical *A*: *My boss will criticize my work.*

Illustrative questions:

- How likely is it that the critical *A* happened (or might happen)?
- Would an objective jury agree that the critical *A* actually happened or might happen? If not, what would the jury's verdict be?
- Did I view (am I viewing) the situation realistically? If not, how could I have viewed (can I view) it more realistically?
- If I asked someone whom I could trust to give me an objective opinion about the truth or falsity of my inference about the situation at hand, what would the person say to me and why? How would this person encourage me to view the situation instead?
- If a friend had told me that they had faced (were facing or were about to face) the same situation as I faced and had made the same inference, what would I say to him/her about the validity of their inference and why? How would I encourage the person to view the situation instead?

Conclusion: *Based on what I know about my boss, the quality of my work that I submitted and what is going on in the company at this time, I think that it is highly unlikely that the reason why my boss wishes to see me is to criticize my work. The most likely explanation is that he wants to discuss aspects of my report in a non-critical way.*

Figure 9.3 Reconsidering the critical *A*: Oliver's example.

- Is my boss generally critical of my work? *No, he does criticize work when it is very sloppy, but he is not generally critical.*
- Have I just handed in work that is very sloppy? *No, the last report that I handed in was quite good. I'm reasonably sure he wouldn't think it sloppy.*
- Have I any other evidence in favour of my inference that the reason that he wants to see me is to criticize my work? *Not that I can think of.*

2 Oliver then considered alternative explanations for his boss requesting to see him. He came up with the following.

- My boss wants to see me to discuss my report in a non-critical way.
- My boss wants to see me to discuss some other aspect of work.

- My boss wants to see me about some non-work issue.
- My boss wants to see me to fire me.

3 Finally, Oliver reviewed the evidence concerning the likelihood of these alternative explanations. In doing so, he took into account his boss's general behaviour, his own work performance and what was going on at work at that time. He took into account that his boss was usually fair minded and non-critical, that there was nothing unusual going on at work and that he was working at a reasonably high standard.

4 After he answered his own questions and reviewed the other alternative explanations for his boss wanting to see him, Oliver was ready to reconsider his critical *A*. He concluded, based on the evidence at hand, that his boss probably wanted to see him to discuss aspects of his report in a non-critical way or some other work-related topic. It turned out that the former was the case.

However, what if the following state of affairs were operative at Oliver's workplace?

1 His boss was generally critical of people's work.
2 Oliver had submitted a piece of work to his boss that was sub-standard.
3 Oliver had criticized his boss at a recent work meeting.

If these conditions existed when Oliver came to reconsider his critical *A* he would likely decide that his original critical *A* was the best bet of all the inferences he had identified, i.e. that his boss would criticize his work as the most likely inference that could be drawn from those available.

Other ways of reconsidering the critical *A* are as follows (these are listed and exemplified in Figure 9.3):

1 How likely is it that the critical *A* happened (or might happen)?
2 Would an objective jury agree that the critical *A* actually happened or might happen? If not, what would the jury's verdict be?
3 Did I view (am I viewing) the situation realistically? If not, how could I have viewed (can I view) it more realistically?
4 If I asked someone whom I could trust to give me an objective opinion about the truth or falsity of my inference about the situation at hand, what would the person say to me and why? How would this person encourage me to view the situation instead?
5 If a friend had told me that they had faced (were facing or were about to face) the same situation as I faced and had made the same inference, what would I say to him/her about the validity of their inference and why? How would I encourage the person to view the situation instead.

11. **Reconsider the critical *A*.** Write down the situation that you listed in step 1 and the critical *A* listed in step 3. Then ask yourself whether or not the critical *A* is the best way of viewing the situation given all the evidence to hand (illustrative questions provided)

    Situation:

    Critical *A*:

Illustrative questions:

- How likely is it that the critical *A* happened (or might happen)?
- Would an objective jury agree that the critical *A* actually happened or might happen? If not, what would the jury's verdict be?
- Did I view (am I viewing) the situation realistically? If not, how could I have viewed (can I view) it more realistically?
- If I asked someone whom I could trust to give me an objective opinion about the truth or falsity of my inference about the situation at hand, what would the person say to me and why? How would this person encourage me to view the situation instead?
- If a friend had told me that they had faced (were facing or were about to face) the same situation as I faced and had made the same inference, what would I say to him/her about the validity of their inference and why? How would I encourage the person to view the situation instead?

Conclusion:

Figure 9.4 Reconsidering *A*.

You are now in a position to reconsider your critical *A* for yourself. Do so in Figure 9.4.

Chapter 10

Improvisations on a theme

I have now shown you how to use the DRF-2. This lengthy form helps you to analyse a situation in which you disturbed yourself. In particular, it helps you to identify your major unhealthy emotion and self-defeating behaviour, what you were most disturbed about, the irrational beliefs that underpinned your disturbed reactions and their healthy alternatives. It further helps you to set goals, question the beliefs that are at the core of your problem and deal with any obstacles to a healthier response that may exist. Finally, it helps you to act on your new healthy belief and to get into the right frame of mind to identify and challenge any distorted inferences you may have made in the first place. In short, the DRF-2 is a comprehensive approach to emotional problem solving.

However, many people complain that the DRF-2 is too long to use at times when a quicker analysis and response is called for. For this reason, I suggest that you devise your own form for use at those times. There is one important point that I want to make before giving you some examples of shortened forms that some of my clients have devised and used for themselves. I strongly suggest that you devise your own shortened forms *after* you have become proficient at using the DRF-2. Why? For the same reason that a jazz player learns how to play his or her instrument proficiently before improvising. Improvisation at REBT is best done after you have developed competence at the basics of REBT.

When you come to devise your own shortened form of the DRF-2, think about which elements of the full form you have found most helpful, and incorporate these into your own form. Remember that you are devising the form for your use alone. If you are consulting an REBT therapist, he or she will help you to devise your own form.

So here are some examples of shortened forms that my clients have devised for themselves.

The first form that I will discuss was devised by Sophie Humphreys, one of my clients, who asked to be mentioned by her real name. She calls the form the 'Shortish Dryden REBT Form' and a worked example appears in Figure 10.1. As you can see the form contains the following elements.

- Description of the situation.
- Identification of the unhealthy negative emotion and behavioural consequences at *C* in the *ABC* framework.
- Identification of the aspect of the situation the person was most disturbed about at *A* (the critical *A*).
- Identification of both healthy and unhealthy beliefs at *B*. Note that Sophie has decided to group 'demands' and 'low frustration tolerance beliefs' together. This is a good example of the idiosyncratic nature of her form in that it suits her to construct it in this way.
- Selection of the emotional and behavioural goals.
- Listing of persuasive arguments to strengthen the conviction in the healthy belief and weaken the conviction in the unhealthy belief.

Shortish Dryden REBT form

1. **Situation**: describe a situation in which I disturbed myself
I called Sarah last night because Molly was driving me mad not going to bed. I decided to leave her, but gave in when she got very distressed. I thought that Sarah thought that I was the problem

2. **C (Consequences)**
Unhealthy negative emotion: *anxiety, depression, shame, guilt, hurt, unhealthy anger, unhealthy jealousy, unhealthy envy*
Behavioural consequences: *became very defensive with Sarah, lied, justified myself, hurt my gums, ran myself down about my appearance.*

3. **Critical *A***: identify the aspect of the situation I was most disturbed about
Not doing the right thing as a mother.

4 ***B* (Beliefs)**

Demand and low frustration tolerance belief =
I must do the right thing as a mother and I can't stand it when I don't

Full preference and high frustration tolerance belief =
I would prefer to do the right thing as a mum but I don't have to do so. It is hard to bear it when I don't do the right thing, but I can bear it and it is worth bearing since doing so will help me to think about how best to address Molly's sleep problem.

Awfulizing belief =
N/A

Anti-awfulizing belief =
N/A

Depreciation belief =
I am a shitty person for not doing the right thing as a mum.

Acceptance belief =
I am not a shitty person for not doing the right thing as a mum. I am a complex, fallible human being who does right and wrong things as a mum.

5. **Choose a healthy alternative to step 2**

Emotional goal: *concern, sadness, disappointment, remorse, sorrow, healthy anger, healthy jealousy, healthy envy*

Behavioural goal: *admit to Sarah that I am having a problem getting Molly off to sleep. Ask her for suggestions about how I might address the problem differently.*

continued . . .

6. **List persuasive arguments that help strengthen my healthy belief and weaken my unhealthy belief**

a) *If there was a law of nature that stated that I must not make any errors as a mother, then I wouldn't be able to. Sadly that's not the case. I can and do make mistakes as a mum and while that's difficult for me to tolerate I can and do tolerate it. If I couldn't bear it, I would have expired well before now.*

b) *By having me as a mother, Molly gets all my good points as well as bad. We're both fallible.*

c)

d)

7. **Respond to any doubts** (about adopting the healthy belief or giving up the unhealthy belief)

Doubt: *But since I am responsible for my daughter's well-being, I mustn't make any errors as a mother.*

Response: *Yes, I am largely responsible for my daughter's well-being but that means that I will do my utmost not to make any errors as a mum. However, I am human and not immune from error. All I can do is my best and learn from any errors I may make.*

Doubt:

Response:

8. **List homework assignments that I can do to strengthen conviction in my healthy belief**

a) *Admit to Sarah that I am having a problem getting Molly off to sleep. Ask her for suggestions about how I might address the problem differently. Do both while reminding myself that I am a fallible human being who would like not to make errors as a mum but is bound to because I'm human.*

b) *While accepting myself as a fallible human being, review on paper my strengths as a mother.*

c)

9. **Reconsider Critical *A*** – did I view it realistically?
I may be doing the wrong thing in trying to get Molly off to sleep or I might be doing the right thing in the wrong way. My frustration may be getting in the way.

Figure 10.1 Shortish Dryden REBT Form.

- Identification and response to doubts about adopting the healthy belief and relinquishing the unhealthy belief.
- Listing of homework assignments to strengthen the conviction in healthy belief.
- Reconsideration of the critical *A*.

The second form that I will discuss is called the 'Quick Dryden REBT Form' (see Figure 10.2) which was also devised by Sophie Humphreys. Sophie constructed this form for use when time is at a premium (i.e. when she does not have the time to fill in her longer, more comprehensive 'Shortish' form) or when she does not need to include all the elements on her 'Shortish' form. As you can see the form contains the following elements.

- Description of the situation and identification of the aspect of the situation that the person was disturbed about. Note that both the situation and the critical *A* are identified here. The critical *A* is highlighted by being underlined.
- Identification of the unhealthy negative emotion and behavioural consequences at *C* in the *ABC* framework.
- Identification of unhealthy beliefs at *B*. Note that Sophie has decided to omit the healthy beliefs here.
- Identification of alternative rational beliefs. Sophie has decided that on this form where time is at a premium, listing the rational beliefs without accompanying arguments is sufficient.
- Identification of new emotional and behavioural consequences of the rational beliefs.

Note that on her 'Quick' form, Sophie has not included the following elements that appear on her 'Shortish' form.

- Identification of the emotional and behavioural goals. Rather, she lists these as new consequences of her rational beliefs.
- Listing of persuasive arguments to strengthen the conviction in the healthy belief and weaken the conviction in the unhealthy belief.
- Identification and response to doubts about adopting the healthy belief and relinquishing the unhealthy belief.
- Listing of homework assignments to strengthen the conviction in the healthy belief.
- Reconsideration of the critical *A*.

Finally, I will discuss the 'Dryden Self-Help Form' (see Figure 10.3) which was devised by another of my clients who wishes to remain anonymous. This form has the following elements.

Quick Dryden REBT form

1. **Activating Event**: describe a situation where I disturbed myself and the aspect of it that I was most disturbed about (underlined)

   Man from sleep clinic did not recognize me with my hair back. I thought that he must think I look ill, therefore maybe I am ill.

2. **Beliefs**: identify irrational beliefs

   Demand and low frustration tolerance: *I must know now for certain that I am not ill and I can't stand not knowing this.*

   Awfulizing belief: *It is awful not knowing for certain that I am not ill.*

   Depreciation belief: N/A

3. **Consequences**

   Unhealthy negative emotion: *anxiety, depression, shame, guilt, hurt, unhealthy anger, unhealthy jealousy, unhealthy envy*

   Behavioural consequences: *Checking, looking in shop window at my reflection, telling people I had a bug last week if they comment on my appearance.*

4. **Rational beliefs**

   Full Preference and high frustration tolerance: *I would prefer to know now that I am not ill but I don't have to know this. I can bear not knowing this and am bearing it. It's worth bearing because it will help me to stop acting in ways that make my hypochondria worse.*

   Anti-awfulizing belief: *It is unfortunate that I don't know for certain that I am not ill but not knowing this is not the end of the world.*

   Acceptance belief: N/A

5. **New Consequences**

   Emotional goal: *concern, sadness, disappointment, remorse, sorrow, healthy anger, healthy jealousy, healthy envy*

   Behavioural goal: *Refraining from acting on my tendency to seek reassurance, refraining from acting on my tendency to look at my reflection in shop windows, just acknowledge what people say about the way I look without adding any explanation.*

Figure 10.2 Quick Dryden REBT Form.

Dryden self-help form

1. **Situation**: *I didn't tell a cyclist that he was riding in a 'No cycling' area.*

2. **Assessment**

A = *I was too scared to say anything to him.*

B = *I absolutely should not have been too scared to say anything. I'm a wimp for being scared.*

C (emotional) = *Anger at self.*

(behavioural) = *Felt like chasing after him and really telling him off.*

3. **Question unhealthy belief** (with healthy belief underlined)

a) *The reality is that I was too scared to say anything and if there was a law that says I absolutely shouldn't have been, I wouldn't have been. But I was, I wish I wasn't, but I was. So, <u>I would have liked not to have been too scared, but I'm not immune from such fear.</u>*

b) *Am I am wimp? No! Sometimes I speak up when I'm scared and sometimes I don't. It doesn't make sense for me to judge my whole self on the basis of one act or even on the basis of a trait. <u>I'm not a wimp. I'm a complex, fallible human being who was too scared on this occasion to speak up.</u>*

4. **Respond to any doubts** (to adopting the healthy belief and relinquishing the unhealthy belief)

Doubt: *But the cyclist was breaking the law. I absolutely shouldn't have let him get away with it.*

Response: *Thank you, Clint Eastwood. This 'come on punk, make my day' macho attitude will get you killed one day if you act on it. Also are you employed by the Council as a one-man upholder of the bye-laws? I may wish I was bigger and stronger but I'm not. I can let these things go without putting myself down.*

5. **New consequences**

Emotional: *Disappointment.*

Behavioural: *Refrain from chasing after cyclist. Let it go.*

6. **Reconsider *A*** (Did I view A realistically?)
A was true. I was too scared to assert myself.

7. **Act on healthy belief to strengthen it**
Walk up and down the promenade while practising my healthy belief and particularly so when I am too scared to tell them about the 'No cycling' law.

Figure 10.3 Dryden Self-Help Form: Example.

- A space for a description of the situation under consideration.
- An assessment section where *ABC* elements are considered together. Note that *C* is divided into emotional and behavioural components. Note also that no guidance is given either about irrational beliefs or what constitute unhealthy negative emotions. As my client said 'I don't need to remind myself of these elements since I am very familiar with them'.
- Spaces for questioning unhealthy beliefs. Note that there is an instruction to list and underline the healthy beliefs.
- Spaces to identify and respond to doubts about adopting the healthy belief and/or giving up the unhealthy belief.
- A space for the new consequences (emotional and behavioural) of the healthy belief.
- A space for the person to reconsider his or her critical *A*.
- A space for the person to detail how he or she is going to strengthen his or her healthy belief in future by acting in a way that is consistent with the healthy belief.

If you want to experiment with using the Dryden Self-Help Form, a blank copy is provided in Figure 10.4.

I have provided a set of instructions in Figure 10.5 to help you use the Dryden Self-Help Form should you wish to do so.

Now it is your turn to devise your own self-help form. If you are consulting an REBT therapist, he or she will give you feedback on your form and help you to refine it.

Dryden self-help form

1. **Situation**:

2. **Assessment**

A =

B =

C (emotional) =

(behavioural) =

3. **Question unhealthy belief** (with healthy belief underlined)

a)

b)

c)

continued . . .

4. **Respond to any doubts** (to adopting the healthy belief and/or relinquishing the unhealthy belief)

Doubt:

Response:

Doubt:

Response:

5. **New consequences**

Emotional:

Behavioural:

6. **Reconsider *A*** (Did I view *A* realistically?)

7. **Act on healthy belief to strengthen it**

Figure 10.4 Dryden Self-Help Form.

Instructions for using the Dryden self-help form

1. **Situation**
   - Write down exactly what happened in the situation in which you disturbed yourself. Be as objective as possible.

2. **Assessment**
   - Begin with *C*.
   - Next to *C* (emotional) write down your most prominent unhealthy negative emotion in the situation under consideration. Choose *one* from the following:

     anxiety
     depression
     shame
     guilt
     hurt
     unhealthy anger
     unhealthy jealousy, or
     unhealthy envy.
   - Next to *C* (behavioural), write down how you acted in the situation under consideration or how you 'felt like' acting.
   - Then go to *A*.
   - Next to *A* write down what you were most disturbed about in the situation under consideration.
   - Finally go to *B*.
   - Next to *B* write down the demand you made about *A* and one of the following irrational beliefs about *A*: an awfulizing belief, a low frustration tolerance or a depreciation belief. Choose the one irrational belief that best accounts for your disturbance.

3. **Question unhealthy belief**
   - Take your unhealthy belief (demand + one other irrational belief from the following: awfulizing belief, LFT belief or depreciation belief) and explain why it is false, illogical and unhelpful.
   - Also state, using underlining, your healthy alternative to this belief.
     This belief will contain a full preference and one other rational belief (anti-awfulizing belief, HFT belief or acceptance belief).

continued . . .

4. **Respond to any doubts**
   - Write down any doubts that you have about adopting your healthy belief and giving up your unhealthy belief.
   - Respond persuasively to these doubts making sure that you deal fully with each one.

5. **New consequences**
   - Write down the healthy consequences of your healthy belief.
   - Next to 'Emotional', write down the healthy alternative to the unhealthy negative emotion that you listed next to *C* (emotional). It will be *one* of the following:

     concern (as the healthy alternative to anxiety)
     sadness (as the healthy alternative to depression)
     disappointment (as the healthy alternative to shame)
     remorse (as the healthy alternative to guilt)
     sorrow (as the healthy alternative to hurt)
     healthy anger (as the healthy alternative to unhealthy anger)
     healthy jealousy (as the healthy alternative to unhealthy jealousy), or
     healthy envy (as the healthy alternative to unhealthy envy).
   - Next to 'Behavioural', write down a more constructive behavioural response to the response you listed under *C* (behavioural).

6. **Reconsider *A***
   - Go back to *A* in step 2 and ask yourself whether or not this was the most accurate way of interpreting what happened in the situation (in step 1). If not, what would be a more realistic way of interpreting what happened?

7. **Act on healthy belief to strengthen it**
   - Write down what you can *do* to strengthen your conviction in your healthy belief underlined in step 3.

Figure 10.5 Instructions for using the Dryden Self-Help Form.

Chapter 11

Dealing with your core unhealthy beliefs

Up to now, I have mainly concentrated on helping you to identify and challenge your specific unhealthy beliefs as they become manifest in specific situations where you disturbed yourself in some way. In this chapter I will help you to identify and deal with your core unhealthy beliefs. A core unhealthy belief (CUB) is a general unhealthy belief that is at the seat of a number of your psychological problems. It has the following features.

1. It is general in nature.
2. It usually relates to a psychological theme such as approval/disapproval, success/failure, certainty/uncertainty, etc.
3. It spans situations that relate to a psychological theme such as rejection. Put another way, you may bring your core unhealthy belief about rejection to a number of situations in which you think you have been or may be rejected.
4. If it involves people it may relate to one person but more often it relates to a number of people.
5. It affects the way you feel, how you behave and how you subsequently think.
6. It has far more dysfunctional than functional consequences, particularly in the longer term.
7. It comprises a demand and at least one of the following: an awfulizing belief, a low frustration tolerance (LFT) belief and a depreciation belief.
8. It leads you to infer the presence of the relevant theme in the absence of corroborative evidence (e.g. you infer that you have been rejected when it is not clear that you have been).

A core healthy belief (CHB) is also a general belief, but it is healthy in nature. If held, it would be the foundation of healthy psychological functioning in response to the negative activating events, about which you presently disturb yourself, related to a psychological theme (e.g. approval/disapproval, success/failure, certainty/uncertainty, etc.). It has all the features of a CUB bar three.

1. It has far more functional than dysfunctional consequences in the longer term.
2. It comprises a full preference and at least one of the following: an anti-awfulizing belief, a high frustration tolerance (HFT) belief and an acceptance belief.
3. It leads you to be accurate in your inferences about the presence or absence of the relevant theme (e.g. you infer that you have been rejected only when it is clear that you have been).

Identifying your core unhealthy beliefs

The following are ways to identify your core unhealthy beliefs.

Examine the critical A's in step 3 of the DRF-2

If you have used the DRF-2 routinely in your self-change programme, you can determine your core unhealthy belief(s) by (a) examining the critical *A*'s you listed in step 3 of the form, (b) seeing if there is a common theme or themes apparent among these critical *A*'s, (c) determining the context(s) in which you disturb yourself related to the theme, (d) determining the range of people involved, if relevant (e.g. authority figures; attractive members of the opposite sex, parents, etc.), and (e) adding the demand and one other irrational belief (i.e. awfulizing belief, LFT belief or depreciation belief) to this theme or themes. Thus, Oliver considered a number of DRF-2 forms that he had completed and discovered that being criticized was a recurring theme and authority figures were the reference group involved at work. Adding the appropriate unhealthy beliefs to this theme yielded the following core unhealthy belief:

> I must not be criticized by authority figures at work and I am an incompetent person if I am criticized by such people.

Identify disturbance-related themes

To identify disturbance-related themes follow these steps.

1 Ask yourself what you largely disturb yourself about from the following list of psychological themes:

being rejected	losing status
failure	acting poorly or foolishly in public
falling short of your ideals	being frustrated
breaking your moral code	discomfort
hurting the feelings of other people	emotional pain
	physical pain
poor performance	loss
being criticized	unfairness/injustice to self
being disapproved of	unfairness/injustice to others
not being loved	being betrayed or let down by others
not being liked	loss of control
someone whom you value preferring someone else to you	uncertainty
	illness
not having something you value which someone else has	loss of security
	physical danger

2 Identify the contexts in which you experience problems related to the identified theme and/or relevant people involved, for example

- theme = being criticized;
- context = at work;
- relevant people = authority figures.

3 Add the demand and at least one other unhealthy belief from the following list: anti-awfulizing belief, LFT belief, depreciation belief (e.g. 'I must not be criticized by authority figures at work and I am an incompetent person if I am criticized by such people').

Monitor your preoccupations

When people are disturbed, they frequently become preoccupied with whatever it is they are disturbed about. Consequently, one way of identifying your core unhealthy beliefs is to make a note of your preoccupations, identify the theme(s) that commonly crop up in them (using the list of themes may help you to do this), identify the relevant context or people (as above) and then add the demand and one other unhealthy belief as before.

Consider what you avoid in life

Another good way to identify your core unhealthy beliefs is to consider what you would go out of your way to avoid in life. Avoidance of situations is often a sure sign that you have a problem, particularly if it is not in your interests to avoid these situations. In considering your avoided situations, identify the theme(s) that link such situations identify the relevant contexts and people involved and then add the belief components as before. For example, Oliver considered that he would go out of his way to avoid (a) being criticized, (b) at work, (c) by authority figures and that when he added the relevant belief components, his core unhealthy belief was 'I must not be criticized by authority figures at work and I am an incompetent person if I am criticized by such people'.

Identify your nightmare scenarios

Quite a powerful way to identify your core unhealthy belief(s) involves you in identifying what I call 'nightmare scenarios'. These are situations that would have you waking up in a cold sweat if you dreamt about them. When you have listed these scenarios follow the steps that I listed above, i.e. identify the theme(s) involved, the contexts/people that are relevant, and add the belief components.

If you have failed to identify any core unhealthy beliefs from the above methods, you may not have any! However, if you suspect that you do, ask someone who knows you very well and whom you trust to help you, or consult an REBT therapist if you are not already doing so.

List your core unhealthy beliefs, their core healthy alternatives and the effects of each

Once you have identified your core unhealthy beliefs, write them down one at a time on a piece of paper and list their effects. These effects are likely to be emotional, behavioural and thinking effects. Then, on the same piece of paper, write down the healthy alternative to each core unhealthy belief (known as the core healthy belief) and list the effects of these healthy beliefs making sure that you provide a constructive effect for every unconstructive effect of the core unhealthy belief. It is important that you list your core healthy beliefs and their effects because you will need to consult this list when you work on changing your CUBs to CHBs.

Figure 11.1 shows the list of core unhealthy beliefs and their effects together with the alternative core healthy beliefs and their effects, as provided by Brenda, one of my clients.

Use the Dryden Core Belief Form (DCBF)

A structured way to change your core unhealthy beliefs involves you using the Dryden Core Belief Form (DCBF), as shown in Figure 11.2, and following its six steps. I will not go into detail about these steps because if you have learned to use the DRF-2, you should find these steps very straightforward.

1 List both your core unhealthy belief (CUB) and its healthy alternative (CHB) in step 1.
2 Select the core belief that you want to strengthen in step 2. If you have elected to strengthen your core unhealthy belief, review the effects of this belief and compare it to the effects that you have listed under your core healthy belief. If you still want to strengthen the core unhealthy belief discuss this with your REBT therapist if you are consulting one, and seek out one for a consultation on this point if you are not (see Appendix 3 for information on how to find an REBT therapist in your area).
3 List the reasons why you want to strengthen this core belief in step 3.
4 Question both beliefs in the same manner that you used to question your specific beliefs in Chapter 6.
5 List and respond to any doubts, reservations and objections to adopting your selected core belief or giving up the other core belief in step 5. Then respond to each expressed doubt, reservation and objection.

Core unhealthy belief	Core healthy belief
1. ***I must have certainty about the safety/health of my loved ones and I can't bear it if I don't.***	1. ***I would prefer to have certainty about the safety/health of my loved ones but I don't need to have it. Not being certain is difficult to bear but I can bear it and it is worth bearing because it will help me to have less anxious relationships with my loved ones.***
Feeling effect	Feeling effect:
* Anxiety	* Concern
Behavioural effects:	Behavioural effects:
* Obsessive checking/telephoning/timing	* Possibly make one phone call – leave message if necessary
* Deliberately avoid getting home before Brian (to avoid having to wait for him)	* Operate on the basis that 'no news means no news' or that it doesn't necessarily mean that there is bad news. Occupy myself after showing myself this
* Going out to look for Brian	* Do a form to reinforce healthy belief rather than going out to look for Brian
Thinking effects:	Thinking effects:
* If I don't have certainty it means that my loved ones are in danger	* Not having certainty does not mean that my loved ones are in danger
* Need for certainty leads me to overestimate the danger/likelihood of disaster	* Not needing certainty does not increase risk to my loved ones
2. ***I must not be alone and it would be terrible if I was.***	2. ***I would much prefer not to be alone, but there's no reason why I absolutely must not be. It would be bad to be alone but not terrible.***
Feeling effect:	Feeling effect:
* Anxiety/afraid of losing my partner	* Concern
Behavioural effects:	Behavioural effects:
* Fuss about Brian's health, making medical appointments for him, vicarious hypochondria	* Stop being hypervigilant about Brian's health. Allow him to be responsible for his health. Stop asking him how he is

continued . . .

* Watch him obsessively on holiday when he goes swimming in the sea	* Don't watch when he is swimming in the sea, read instead
* Prevent him from going cycling/scuba diving	* Allow him to go scuba diving and cycling in the countryside, but not in Central London. Develop and pursue own hobbies
* Discourage him from going abroad on business trips	* Allow him to go abroad on business trips
* Accompany him to shops/on errands when I don't really want to go	* Go shopping with him only when I want to and not when I am anxious
Thinking effects:	Thinking effects:
* I could not enjoy myself if I were alone	* I could enjoy myself if I were alone, but I would probably enjoy myself more with a partner
* I have been a part of a couple all my adult life, I do not know how to be alone	* I could learn how to be alone although it might be difficult
* I would lose everything if I were alone	* If I am alone, I would have lost a hell of a lot, but not everything, I will still have friends, skills and interests
3. ***I must have a marriage free from strife and tension and I couldn't bear not having this.***	3. ***I would much prefer to have a stress-free marriage but I don't have to have this. It's hard to bear marital strife, but I can bear it and it is worth bearing because it will help me to address rather than avoid problems.***
Feeling effects:	Feeling effects:
* Anxiety	* Concern
* Unhealthy anger (unexpressed)	* Healthy anger (expressed)
Behavioural effects:	Behavioural effects:
* Take every possible step to avoid Brian becoming stressed (do chores myself, ensure that we don't run out of things, ensure that his shirts are ironed and suits dry cleaned)	* Cut down on the amount I do for Brian to a reasonable level and encourage him to do things for himself
* Plead with him when he becomes stressed (this only leads to rows and more stress)	* When he is stressed leave him to cool down on his own

continued . . .

* Nag him to seek therapy and constantly check to see if he has	* Calmly encourage him to seek therapy but leave that decision up to him and don't check
Thinking effects:	Thinking effects:
* Think that a little stress will lead very quickly to a lot	* See that a little stress does not inevitably lead to a lot and that stress dealt with thoughtfully is less stressful than stress dealt with in anxious desperation to get rid of it quickly
* It is my responsibility to deal with stress in the marriage	* It is our joint responsibility to deal with marital strife
4 ***I must succeed in my business life and if I don't I am a failure.***	4. ***I want to succeed in my business life but I don't have to do so. If I don't succeed, I am not a failure; I am a fallible human being who has many different aspects and interests, far too many to be defined by not succeeding at work.***
Feeling effects:	Feeling effects:
* Anxiety	* Concern
* Depression	* Sadness/Disappointment
Behavioural effects:	Behavioural effects:
* Stay late at the office every night	* Stay late at the office only when it is really important and healthy for me to so
* Comply with unreasonable requests in order to earn brownie points	* Say no to unreasonable requests
* Work over the weekends	* Play and relax over the weekends
* Only read work-related books	* Read for pleasure and fun
Thinking effects:	Thinking effects:
* Think about work for much of the time	* Think about a variety of topics including, but not exclusively, work
* Think that time spent not working is a waste of time	* Think that time spent not working is time well spent
* Think that people will not like me if I am not successful at work	* Think that people will like or dislike me for a variety of reasons and while some will not like me if I am not successful at work, most won't care much about this

Figure 11.1 Brenda's core beliefs and their effects.

The Dryden core belief form (DCBF)

1. List your core unhealthy belief in the form of a demand and one of the following irrational beliefs: awfulizing belief, low frustration tolerance belief or depreciation belief. Then list next to it your alternative core healthy belief in the form of a full preference and one of the following rational beliefs: anti-awfulizing belief, high frustration tolerance belief or acceptance belief.

   Core unhealthy belief (CUB) **Core healthy belief (CHB)**

2. Select the core belief that you wish to strengthen.

3. Explain why you wish to strengthen it.

   i)

   ii)

   iii)

   iv)

   v)

continued . . .

4. List persuasive arguments that would help you to strengthen your conviction in your chosen core belief and weaken your conviction in the other core belief (see step 1).

   i)

   ii)

   iii)

   iv)

   v)

   vi)

   vii)

   viii)

   ix)

continued . . .

5. List any doubts, reservations and objections you have about adopting your selected core belief or giving up the other core belief. Then respond to each doubt, reservation or objection.

   a) Doubt, reservation, objection:

      Response:

   b) Doubt, reservation, objection:

      Response:

   c) Doubt, reservation, objection:

      Response:

   d) Doubt, reservation, objection:

      Response:

   e) Doubt, reservation, objection:

      Response:

continued . . .

6. List homework assignments that you can do to strengthen your conviction in your selected core belief and weaken your conviction in the other core belief. Choose assignments where you act and think in ways that are consistent with your selected core belief and inconsistent with the other core belief.

   i)

   ii)

   iii)

   iv)

   v)

   vi)

   vii)

   viii)

Figure 11.2 Dryden Core Belief Form (DCBF)

6 Finally, and perhaps most importantly, in step 6 list homework assignments to help you to strengthen your conviction in your selected core belief and weaken your conviction in the other core belief. As you do so, bear in mind the following points:

- It is important that you practise your healthy core belief while acting and thinking in ways that are consistent with this belief. If you are unsure about this write down the constructive behavioural and thinking effects that stem from the core healthy belief that you wish to strengthen, as listed on your core belief sheet (re-read Figure 11.1 for an example of this sheet).
- Conversely, refrain from acting and thinking in ways that are consistent with your old core unhealthy belief. This will be difficult for you because you are used to acting and thinking in unconstructive ways when your core unhealthy belief is activated. However, if you monitor your belief, your behaviour and your subsequent thinking, and respond constructively to all three when you identify them, then you will go against your tendency to evaluate yourself, others and/or the world in rigid and extreme terms (belief), to act self-defeatingly (behaviour) and to think unrealistically (subsequent thinking) and you will gain valuable experience at weakening your conviction in your core unhealthy beliefs and strengthen your conviction in your core healthy beliefs.
- You will experience a change in your unhealthy negative emotions after much integrated practice at holding on to your core healthy belief and acting and thinking in ways that are consistent with this belief. Thus, emotional change tends to lag behind behavioural change and thinking change. If you understand this, then you will persist at changing your thinking and behaviour and not get discouraged when your feelings take a longer time to change.
- It is important that you face negative events about which you have a problem so that you can practise your core healthy belief and the constructive thinking and acting that stem from this belief. As you do so, I suggest that you expose yourself to events that pose a challenge to your developing core healthy belief and related thoughts and behaviour, but which you do not find overwhelming for you at that time.

  Thus, if you are endeavouring to practise your core healthy belief 'I want to be approved by significant others, but it's not essential that I receive such approval. I am not an unlikeable person. I am a fallible person who can be approved and disapproved', it is important that you review this belief in the face of lack of approval or active disapproval from others. It would be helpful to draw up a hierarchy of people that you think may not approve of you and may even disapprove of you. Here is an example of such a hierarchy based on the 'challenging but not overwhelming' principle (lower items on the hierarchy are 'easier' for the person than higher items):

a) telling my parents that I am gay
b) telling my boss at work that I disagree with working practices
c) telling my friend that he has body odour
d) showing my boss work that he might criticize
e) disagreeing with my parents about politics
f) telling my friends that I am not interested in football
g) complaining about service at my local restaurant and going back
h) taking goods back to a shop that I am unhappy with.

It is important to realize that the person in the above example confronted each situation while reviewing his core healthy belief (tailored for each situation), and while acting in ways that are consistent with this belief. He also put in place a strategy of identifying and responding to instances when he returned his old core unhealthy belief, his unhealthy ways of acting and thinking which stemmed from the core unhealthy belief.

Figure 11.3 gives an example of how one of my clients completed the DCBF.

The Dryden core belief form (DCBF)

1. **List your core unhealthy belief in the form of a demand and one of the following irrational beliefs: awfulizing belief, low frustration tolerance belief or depreciation belief. Then list next to it your alternative core healthy belief in the form of a full preference and one of the following rational beliefs: anti-awfulizing belief, high frustration tolerance belief or acceptance belief.**

Core unhealthy belief (CUB)	**Core healthy belief (CHB)**
I must please people in authority and I can't stand it if I don't	*I'd rather please people in authority but I don't have to do so. It's hard to tolerate not pleasing authority figures but I can stand it.*

2. **Select the core belief that you wish to strengthen.**

I'd rather please people in authority, but I don't have to do so. It's hard to tolerate not pleasing authority figures but I can stand it.

continued . . .

3. Explain why you wish to strengthen it.

i) *This belief will help me to become far less tense at work.*

ii) *This belief will help me to take healthy risks at work.*

iii) *This belief will help me to disagree with authority figures when there is no real risk in doing so and to stop acting in an obsequious manner.*

iv) *This belief will help me to stop thinking about what I think authority figures want me to do and will help me to focus on what I want to do.*

4. List persuasive arguments that would help you to strengthen your conviction in your chosen core belief and weaken your conviction in the other core belief (see step 1).

i) *My core healthy belief (CHB) is consistent with reality because while it is true that I'd rather please authority figures, there is no law of the universe decreeing that I must do so. If there was then I would always please them no matter what I did.*

ii) *I can tolerate authority figures being displeased with me even when I think that I can't tolerate it.*

iii) *If I couldn't tolerate displeasing authority figures then I would have died by now. I would also have lost my capability to be happy. Neither of these things has happened nor, in all probability, will they happen.*

iv) *While I want to please authority figures it doesn't follow logically that I must do so.*

v) *While it is difficult for me to tolerate not pleasing authority figures, it doesn't follow logically that I can't do so.*

vi) *Not only can I bear not pleasing authority figures, it is worth it for me to do so because it will lead me to be more relaxed around them and to be more myself in their company.*

vii) *My core unhealthy belief (CUB) is guaranteed to lead me to be anxious in the company of authority figures. It will also lead me to conform to what I think they want me to do, so that I will be outer directed rather than inner directed.*

viii) *My CUB doesn't make sense because it implies that it is necessary for me not to displease authority figures when this is only my preference. It also implies that because it is hard for me to tolerate displeasing people in authority, doing so is intolerable. This again doesn't follow logically.*

5. List any doubts, reservations and objections you have about adopting your selected core belief or giving up the other core belief. Then respond to each doubt, reservation or objection.

a) Doubt, reservation, objection: *If I adopt my core healthy belief (CHB) I will increase the chances of getting into trouble with authority figures.*
Response: *This may well be true but it will be worth it because I will be more genuine in my dealings with them. Before they only were pleased with me when I put on an act.*

continued . . .

b) Doubt, reservation, objection: *I'll be more anxious if I adopt my CHB because I will be disagreeing with authority figures more.*
Response: If I really adopt my CHB, then I won't feel anxious about disagreeing with authority figures. I'll feel concerned rather than anxious about this and this will be a healthy response.

c) Doubt, reservation, objection: *My core unhealthy belief (CUB) has helped me to get on and without it I won't do as well in my career.*
Response: *It is true that I have done well in my career and it may well be the case that pleasing authority figures at work has helped me to do this. But giving up my CUB doesn't mean that I will stop pleasing work authority figures. It means that I will give up needing to do so and give up always doing so in practice. In any case, many people get on in their careers without being 'yes men' or 'yes women'.*

d) Doubt, reservation, objection: *If I speak my mind then authority figures are bound to be angry with me and I couldn't bear that.*
Response: *First of all, speaking my mind will not automatically lead to authority figures being angry with me although my CUB will lead me to think so. If some of them do get angry with me that's uncomfortable but I certainly could bear it.*

6. List homework assignments that you can do to strengthen your conviction in your selected core belief and weaken your conviction in the other core belief. Choose assignments where you act and think in ways that are consistent with your selected core belief and inconsistent with the other core belief.

i) *I'll give my opinions in meetings at work and risk my boss being displeased with me. Before I do this, while doing it and after doing it I'll rehearse my core health belief (CHB). I will do this rehearsal in all the following assignments.*

ii) *I'll stop being obsequious with the directors when they visit my office, and when they ask me if everything is OK in the office I will mention one or two things that aren't going well when I know this isn't what they want to hear.*

iii) *I'll disagree with my father rather than agreeing with him or staying silent.*

iv) *I'll tell my father that my wife and I will be going abroad this Christmas and won't be visiting him and his wife.*

v) *I won't volunteer for any more extra duties on the Church committee and if the vicar asks me to take them on I will decline to do them. I'll remind myself that the vicar seems to accept it when other committee members decline to do more for the Church so it is unlikely that he'll get cross with me.*

Figure 11.3 Dryden Core Belief Form (DCBF): an example

Keep going when the going gets tough

In Chapter 8 I reviewed the obstacles that you might encounter when you carry out homework assignments based on strengthening your conviction in your specific healthy beliefs, and I suggested ways of overcoming such obstacles. I suggest that you re-read this material now because it is also relevant when considering blocks to carrying out homework assignments that are designed to strengthen your conviction in your core healthy beliefs, and how best to address these blocks. Rather than repeat myself here, I will suggest several broad principles to bear in mind when attempting to change core unhealthy beliefs.

1 Changing core unhealthy beliefs is difficult and requires persistence.
2 As you act in ways that are consistent with your newly developing core healthy beliefs, you will encounter discomfort. It is important to tolerate this discomfort and go forward.
3 The change process is rarely smooth. Accept this grim reality and go forward nevertheless.
4 If something that you do doesn't work, don't awfulize about this. Stand back and learn from it.
5 Accept yourself when you fail at something or when you don't make progress as quickly as you'd like. It may be that you are doing something to slow up the process of change and if so, accept responsibility for this, learn from it and correct it. Depreciating yourself will only slow up the process of change even more.

If you are consulting an REBT therapist, discuss obstacles to core belief change and how to overcome them with him/her. If you are using this workbook on your own and you get stuck at this point, it may be useful to discuss this with an REBT therapist for a session or two (see Appendix 3) before going back to using this material on your own.

Chapter 12

Strengthening your conviction in your core and specific healthy beliefs

In the previous chapter I stressed the importance of thinking and acting in consistent ways if you are to change core unhealthy beliefs. In this chapter I will teach you a number of techniques devised to help you strengthen your conviction in your healthy beliefs and weaken your conviction in your unhealthy beliefs. But why should you need to strengthen your conviction in your healthy beliefs? Why isn't understanding that they are consistent with reality, logical and helpful to you sufficient to bring about change? This latter form of understanding is known as *intellectual insight* and when you have it you say things such as 'I understand why my healthy belief is healthy, but I don't believe it yet' or 'I understand that my healthy belief is healthy up here' (referring to your head) 'but not down here' (referring to your gut). This type of insight is necessary to help you change your core and specific unhealthy beliefs, but it is not sufficient for you to make the change.

The type of insight that does promote change is known by REBT therapists as *emotional insight*. If you had this type of insight you would say such things as 'not only do I believe it in my head, I feel it in my gut' and 'I really believe in my heart that my healthy belief is true, logical and helpful'. The true indicator of whether you have emotional insight into your core and specific healthy beliefs is that this belief leads to healthy emotions, constructive behaviour and realistic thinking. The most powerful way of achieving such emotional insight is repeated practice at holding healthy beliefs, and acting and thinking in ways that are consistent with these beliefs. There are other techniques to promote emotional insight through strengthening your conviction in your healthy beliefs, and these techniques are described in this chapter. Most of these techniques can be used to strengthen your conviction in both your core and your specific healthy beliefs, unless otherwise specified. As before I will describe the technique and show how one of my clients used it for themselves.

Using the rational portfolio method

The rational portfolio method requires you to develop a portfolio of arguments, some of which support your core or specific healthy belief while others contradict your core or specific unhealthy belief. What follows is a set of instructions for its use.

Instructions on how to use the rational portfolio method

1 Take one of your core or specific unhealthy beliefs and the healthy alternative to this belief. Your unhealthy belief should include a demand

and one of the following beliefs (an awfulizing belief, a low frustration tolerance (LFT) belief or a depreciation belief).

2 Write each belief on a separate piece of paper under the appropriate heading:

- specific or core unhealthy belief, and
- specific or core healthy belief.

3 Take your specific or core unhealthy belief and write down as many persuasive arguments you can think of against this unhealthy belief. Remember that such beliefs are

- inconsistent with reality or false;
- illogical;
- generally yield poor results.

You might find it useful to consult the material I presented in Chapter 6 as you develop your list of arguments.

4 Next, take your specific or core healthy belief and write down as many persuasive arguments as you can think of that support this healthy belief. Remember that such beliefs are

- consistent with reality or true;
- logical;
- generally yield good results.

Once again you might find it useful to consult the material I presented in Chapter 6 as you develop your list of arguments.

5 Review this list regularly adding persuasive arguments to each list as you think of them.

A rational portfolio compiled by one of my clients is shown in the box below.

Heather's rational portfolio

Core unhealthy belief

People that I have just met must like me and if they don't it means that I am an unlikeable person.

Reasons why this core belief is unhealthy

- There is no law of the universe that states that new people must like me. If there was such a law then they would have to like me no matter how I treated them.
- When I demand that new people must like me, I am depriving them of the freedom to dislike me or to be neutral to me. My demand deprives them of free will.
- Even if new people are wrong not to like me when they first meet me, my demand deprives them of their right to be wrong. Hence my demand is dogmatic and fascistic.
- Even if I go out of my way to be friendly to people that I have just met, they don't all have to like me. People are very different and some will dislike me for the very reason that I am, in their eyes, overly friendly with them.
- If someone that I have just met dislikes me or is neutral towards me then this is a fact. When I demand that the person must like me I am in fact demanding that reality must not be the way that it is; rather, it must be the way that I want it to be. That would be fine if I ran the universe, but clearly I don't.
- I don't like every new person that I meet therefore why must all new people like me? Obviously they don't.
- It would be nice if everyone that I met were to like me but it is illogical for me to conclude that it must be that way. The first part of that statement is flexible and the second part is rigid and one cannot logically derive something rigid from something flexible.
- As long as I demand that people that I have just met must like me, I will be anxious in case they don't.
- If I demand that people that I have just met must like me, I will be anxious even if they do like me, because they may change their mind later.
- If I demand that new people must like me, I will assume that they don't like me if they give me a neutral response.
- If I demand that new people must like me, then this demand will lead me to try desperately to get them to like me. When I act desperately and people like me for it then they will tend to like me for the image that I portray and I will remain anxious in case they don't like me when I reveal the real me.
- When I conclude that I am an unlikeable person if people I have just met do not like me, I am saying that there is nothing likeable about me. For this is what being an unlikeable person means. This is not

true since there are things that are both likeable and unlikeable about me.

- When I say that I am an unlikeable person if people I have just met dislike me, then I am implying that I can be rated as a person. This is not true since I am a complex, everchanging fallible human being and while aspects of myself can legitimately be rated, my 'self' cannot be.
- If new people dislike me when they first meet me, this is hardly evidence that I am an unlikeable person, not capable of being liked. If it means anything, it may mean that I behave in a way that puts people off me. If this is the case it doesn't prove that I am unlikeable. It means that I am a fallible human being who is acting poorly.
- If people I have just met dislike me then this may say something about their preferences. My worth cannot be based on other people's preferences.
- When I rate myself as an unlikeable person based on people I have just met not liking me, I am making an illogical overgeneralization, for I am saying because it is bad if they don't like me then this badness proves that I am unlikeable. Also, even if I have a dislikeable trait which turns off people I have just met, it is also illogical for me to conclude that I am an unlikeable person because of such a trait.
- If I think that I am unlikeable person if people I have just met do not like me, then I will be anxious before meeting them and when I am talking to them because there is always a chance of them not liking me. This belief will also lead me to be depressed after meeting them if I think that they don't like me.
- When I think that I am an unlikeable person if new people do not like me, this belief will lead me to overestimate in my mind the probability that they will not like me.
- When I think that I am unlikeable person if new people do not like me, I will be sceptical if they show that they like me. I may think that they feel sorry for me or that they have an ulterior motive for being friendly.
- If I think that I am unlikeable person if new people do not like me, I will tend to avoid meeting new people or withdraw from social gatherings where there are strangers as quickly as I can. Thus, I deprive myself of much pleasure.
- If new people show that they like me, I may wrongly conclude that I am a likeable person setting myself up to believe that I am unlikeable if they or others don't show that they like me later. I thus reinforce my philosophy that my likeability as a person is based on others' actual or presumed responses to me when I first met them.

Core healthy belief

I want people that I have just met to like me, but they don't have to like me. If they don't it doesn't mean that I am an unlikeable person. It means that I am a fallible human being capable of being liked and disliked.

Reasons why this core belief is healthy

- My full preference is true because I am indicating the truth of my desire, that is, I want people that I have just met to like me.
- My full preference is also true because I acknowledge that there is no law of the universe that states that people I have just met must like me.
- By wanting new people to like me, but by not demanding that they have to, I am acknowledging that they have the freedom to dislike me or be neutral to me if this is how they feel towards me.
- My acknowledgement that people that I have just met don't have to like me (flexible statement) follows logically from my flexible desire that I want them to like me.
- If new people don't like me then this is a fact and when I state that I want them to like me, but don't demand that they have to do so, I am acknowledging that reality does not have to be the way that I want it to be.
- Wanting new people to like me but not demanding that they have to do so will lead me to be concerned, but not anxious, over the possibility that they might not like me and sad, but not depressed, once it becomes clear that they don't like me. Concern and sadness are healthy negative emotions because they help me to face up to a negative situation without disturbing myself about it.
- When I want new people to like me, but don't demand that they have to do so, this belief will lead me to be friendly towards them without desperately trying to get them to like me. This approach will increase rather than decrease the chances that they will like me and like me for myself rather than for any act that I put on.
- If new people like me, then my full preference will lead me to be concerned rather than anxious about the possibility that they may dislike me later.
- When I want new people to like me, but do not demand that they have to do so, I will not automatically assume that they don't like me unless I have clear evidence to this effect. I will allow for the possibility that they may like me or feel neutral towards me.

- When I conclude that I am a fallible human being capable of being liked and disliked if new people don't like me, I am making a true statement.
- If new people don't like me and this is because of my dislikeable behaviour or a dislikeable trait, this only proves that I am a fallible human being who has acted in a dislikeable manner or has a dislikeable trait. It does not prove that I am a dislikeable person.
- If new people don't like me, they may be saying more about their preferences about people than about me as a person. The fact that I am a fallible human being capable of being liked and disliked is true, no matter what their preferences are.
- When I conclude that I am a fallible human being capable of being liked and disliked when new people dislike me, this is a logical conclusion. I am not making the part–whole error when I make such a conclusion.
- When I accept myself as a fallible human being capable of being liked and disliked, I will be concerned but not anxious if there is a possibility that new people may dislike me.
- When I accept myself as a fallible human being capable of being liked and disliked, I will be sad, but not depressed, if it is clear that they don't like me.
- When I accept myself as a fallible human being capable of being liked and disliked, I will not tend to conclude that people I have just met will dislike me. I will acknowledge that they will have a range of responses towards me and will make any decision about their attitude towards me on the basis of evidence.
- When I accept myself as a fallible human being capable of being liked and disliked, I will take new people's friendliness towards me at face value and not think that they feel sorry for me or have an ulterior motive for their friendliness.
- If I accept myself as fallible human being capable of being liked and disliked, I will not avoid meeting new people in social situations.
- If I accept myself as fallible human being capable of being liked and disliked, I will not withdraw from social situations when some new people show that they dislike me.
- If I accept myself as fallible human being capable of being liked and disliked, I will not stay silent when meeting new people. I will talk to them and voice my opinions.
- If new people show that they like me, I will not regard myself as a likeable person. I will still see myself as a fallible human being capable of being liked and disliked. My attitude towards myself will not fluctuate according to whether new people like me or not.

Using zig-zag techniques

You may find as you embark on the process of strengthening your conviction in your healthy beliefs (whether they be core or specific) that you will counteract this process in your head. In Chapter 7 I have already discussed how to identify and deal with your doubts, reservations and objections to adopting healthy beliefs. In this chapter I will describe two zig-zag techniques which capitalize on your tendency to 'attack' your core and/or specific healthy beliefs and encourage you to respond to these attacks as a way of strengthening your conviction in your healthy beliefs. Here, I will teach you how to use the written zig-zag form (see Figure 12.1) and the tape-recorded version of the zig-zag technique.

Instructions on how to complete a written zig-zag form

1. Write down your core or specific healthy belief in the top left-hand box.
2. Rate your present level of conviction in this belief on a 100 per cent point scale where 0 per cent is no conviction and 100 per cent is total conviction (i.e. you really believe it in your heart and it markedly influences your feelings and behaviour). Write down this rating in the space provided on the form.
3. Attack this healthy belief. Your attack may take the form of a doubt, reservation or objection to this healthy belief. It should also contain an explicit irrational belief (e.g. demand, awfulizing belief, LFT belief or depreciating belief). Make this attack as genuinely as you can. The more it reflects what you believe, the better. Write down this attack in the first box on the right.
4. Respond to this attack as fully as you can. It is really important that you respond to each element of the attack. In particular, make sure that you respond to unhealthy belief statements and also to distorted or unrealistic inferences framed in the form of a doubt, reservation or objection to the healthy belief. Do so as persuasively as possible and write down your response in the second box on the left.
5. Continue in this vein until you have answered all of your attacks and cannot think of any more. Make sure throughout this process that you are keeping the focus on the healthy belief that you are trying to strengthen.

If you find this exercise difficult, you might find it easier to make your attacks gently at first. Then, when you find that you can respond to these attacks quite easily, begin to make the attacks more biting. Work in this way until you are making really strong attacks. When you make an attack, do so as if you really want to believe it. And when you respond, really throw yourself into it with the intention of demolishing the attack and of strengthening your conviction in your healthy belief.

Don't forget that the purpose of this exercise is to strengthen your conviction in your healthy belief, so it is important that you stop only when you have answered all of your attacks. Use as many forms as you need and clip them together when you have finished.

If you make an attack that you cannot respond to, stop the exercise and raise the issue with your REBT therapist if you are consulting one, or if you are using this workbook on your own discuss the attack with a friend who may be able to give you some ideas about how best to respond to it.

6 When you have answered all of your attacks, re-rate your level of conviction in your healthy belief using the 0–100 per cent scale as before. If you have succeeded at responding persuasively to your attacks, then this rating will have gone up appreciably. If it has not increased, has only increased a little, or has gone down, do the following.
7 Re-read what you have written and note:

- instances when you went off the point, formulate an alternative response at this point that would have enabled you to keep to the point;
- instances when you failed to respond to an element (or elements) of an attack (in particular an unrealistic or distorted inference or an unhealthy belief statement), formulate a response to that unanswered element (or elements);
- instances when you were unpersuaded by your response to an attack, formulate more persuasive ways of responding to this attack in both use of language and content of argument.

You could also discuss these issues with your REBT therapist or with a friend.

Figure 12.2 shows how one person used the written zig-zag form to strengthen her conviction in a specific healthy belief.

Once you have become proficient at using the written zig-zag form, you can move on to using the tape-recorded zig-zag technique. The purpose of this variation is the same as in the written zig-zag: to strengthen your conviction in your developing core and/or specific healthy beliefs by responding persuasively to attacks on them. However, as you use spoken language in this variation (as opposed to written language in the written version of the zig-zag), you can use your voice tone and the forcefulness of your spoken words to aid you in this process. Indeed, as you use the tape-recorded zig-zag, make sure that the force and tone of your voice is more persuasive and your language is more evocative when responding to attacks on your healthy beliefs than when making these attacks. With this important consideration in mind, this is how to use the tape-recorded zig-zag.

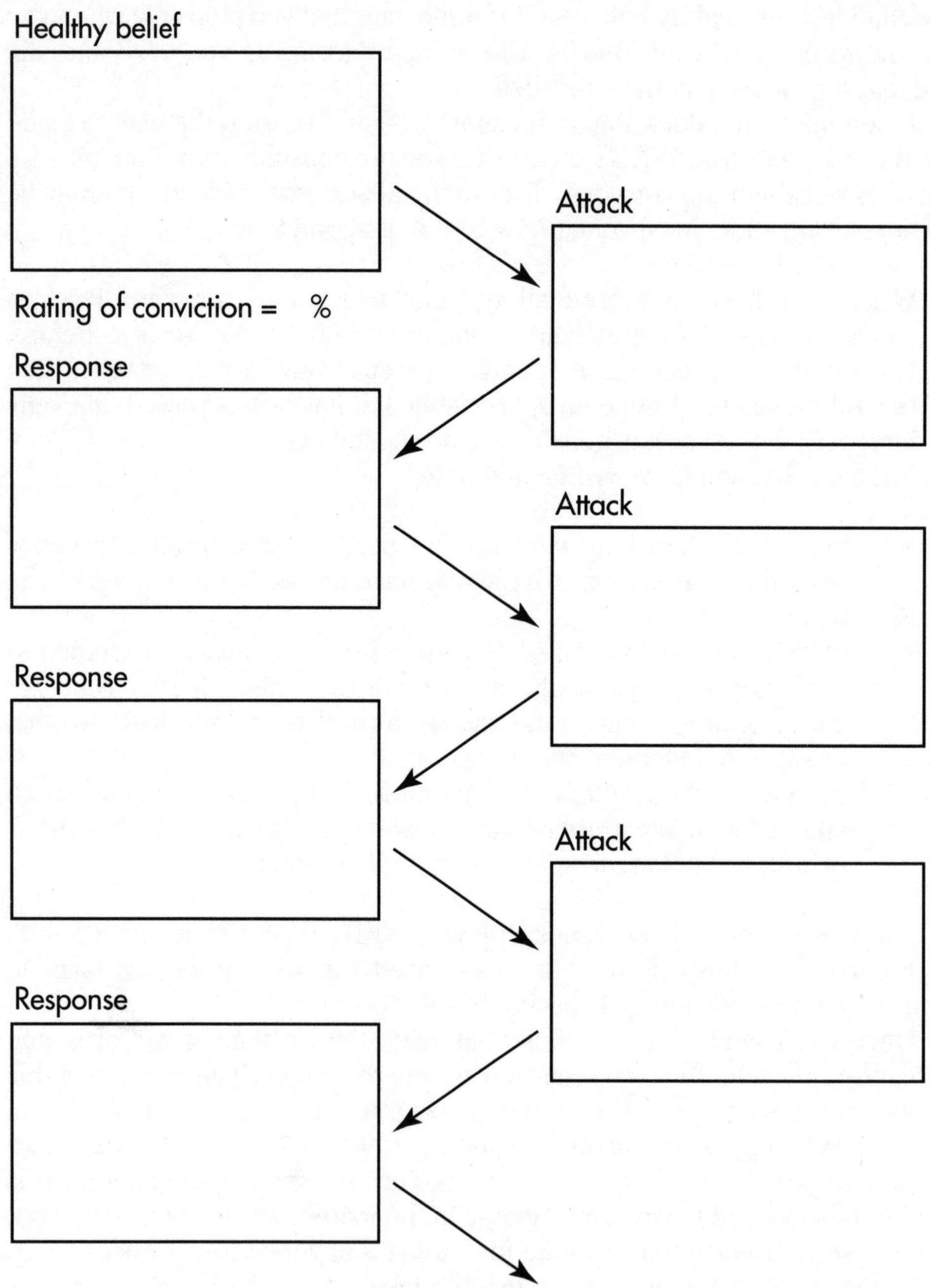
Healthy belief
Attack
Rating of conviction = %
Response
Attack
Response
Attack
Response

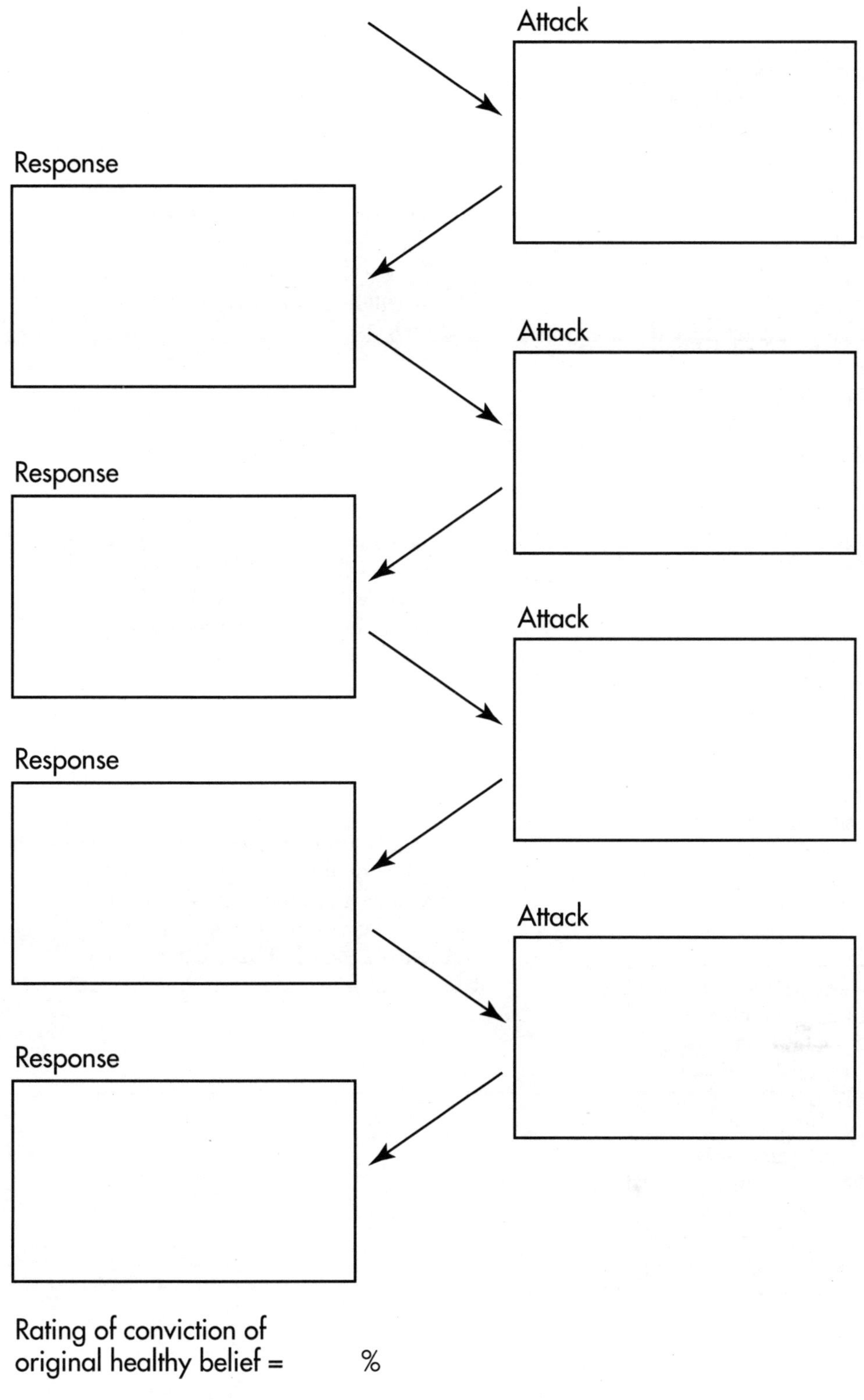

Rating of conviction of original healthy belief = %

Figure 12.1 Zig-zag form.

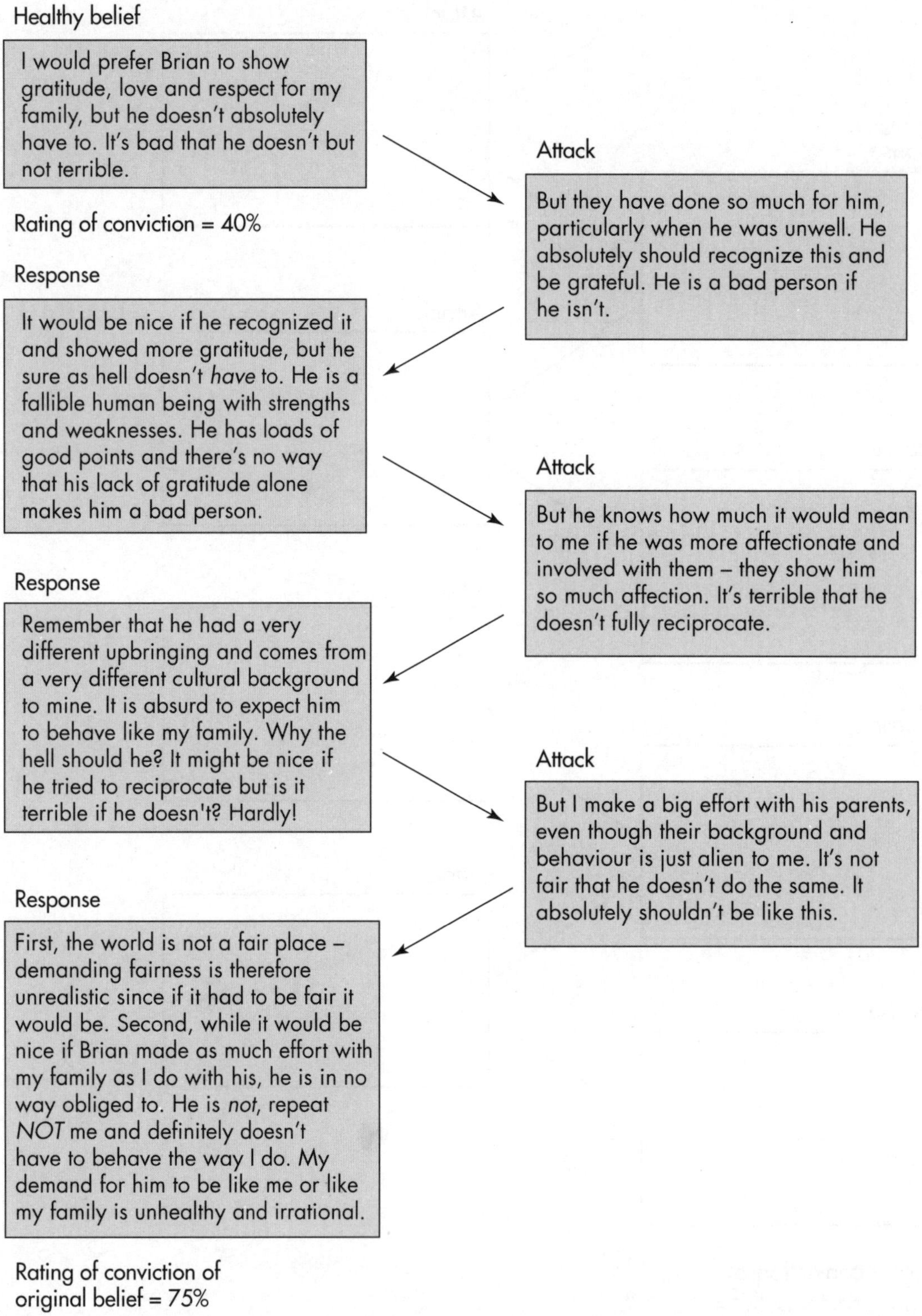

Healthy belief

I would prefer Brian to show gratitude, love and respect for my family, but he doesn't absolutely have to. It's bad that he doesn't but not terrible.

Rating of conviction = 40%

Attack

But they have done so much for him, particularly when he was unwell. He absolutely should recognize this and be grateful. He is a bad person if he isn't.

Response

It would be nice if he recognized it and showed more gratitude, but he sure as hell doesn't *have* to. He is a fallible human being with strengths and weaknesses. He has loads of good points and there's no way that his lack of gratitude alone makes him a bad person.

Attack

But he knows how much it would mean to me if he was more affectionate and involved with them – they show him so much affection. It's terrible that he doesn't fully reciprocate.

Response

Remember that he had a very different upbringing and comes from a very different cultural background to mine. It is absurd to expect him to behave like my family. Why the hell should he? It might be nice if he tried to reciprocate but is it terrible if he doesn't? Hardly!

Attack

But I make a big effort with his parents, even though their background and behaviour is just alien to me. It's not fair that he doesn't do the same. It absolutely shouldn't be like this.

Response

First, the world is not a fair place – demanding fairness is therefore unrealistic since if it had to be fair it would be. Second, while it would be nice if Brian made as much effort with my family as I do with his, he is in no way obliged to. He is *not*, repeat *NOT* me and definitely doesn't have to behave the way I do. My demand for him to be like me or like my family is unhealthy and irrational.

Rating of conviction of original belief = 75%

Figure 12.2 Zig-zag technique: an example

Instructions on how to use the tape-recorded version of the zig-zag technique

1. You will need to use a hand-held, good-quality recorder with a good-quality tape for this exercise. A good micro- or mini-cassette recorder will suffice.
2. Find a time and a place where you won't be interrupted and cannot be overheard. Put your answer machine on or take the phone off the hook. You will need to set aside about 20 to 30 minutes for this task.
3. Begin the recording process by stating your healthy belief on tape and noting verbally your level of conviction in it, using the 0–100 per cent scale.
4. Try and get yourself to return to your unhealthy belief by attacking your healthy belief on tape using doubts, reservations or objections to this belief and associated unhealthy belief statements.
5. Respond to this attack on tape in a forceful and persuasive manner making sure that you answer all elements of this attack. In particular respond to the unrealistic aspects of the doubts, reservations and objections, and to the associated unhealthy belief statements.
6. Go back and forth in this manner (making sure that your responses are more forceful and persuasive than your attacks) until you can no longer think of any attacks. Make sure throughout this process that you are keeping the focus on the healthy belief that you are trying to strengthen.
7. Re-rate your level of conviction in your originally stated healthy belief and state this on the tape. If you have succeeded in responding persuasively to your attacks, then the rating will have gone up appreciably. If it has not increased, has only increased a little, or has gone down, do the following.
8. Listen to the recording and note:

    - instances when you went off the point, formulate an alternative response at this point that would have enabled you to keep to the point;
    - instances when you failed to respond to an element (or elements) of an attack (in particular an unrealistic or distorted inference or an unhealthy belief statement), formulate a response to that unanswered element (or elements);
    - instances when you sounded unpersuaded by your response to an attack, formulate more persuasive ways of responding to this attack in tone of voice, use of language and content of argument.

Once again you could discuss these issues with your REBT therapist or with a friend.

Using rational-emotive imagery

Rational-emotive imagery (REI) is an imagery method designed to help you practise changing your *specific* unhealthy belief to its healthy equivalent while you imagine, at the same time, focusing on what you are most disturbed about in a *specific* situation in which you felt disturbed. Because you can only use REI while imagining specific situations, it is recommended for use only to strengthen your conviction in *specific* healthy beliefs. There are two versions of rational-emotive imagery, one devised by Dr Albert Ellis, the originator of REBT, and the other devised by Dr Maxie C. Maultsby Jr. I will teach you the Ellis version first and then the Maultsby technique. I suggest that you use both techniques for a time to determine which is more effective for you.

You can use your imagery modality to help you get over your problems, or to, albeit unwittingly, practise thinking unhealthily as you imagine a host of negative situations about which you disturb yourself. In the latter case, when you think about a negative event and you disturb yourself about it, you are likely to do so by imagining the event in your mind's eye and covertly rehearsing one or more unhealthy beliefs about the event. In this way, you literally practise disturbing yourself and at the same time you end up by strengthening your conviction in your unhealthy beliefs.

Fortunately you can also use your mind's eye for constructive purposes. For instance, while imagining the same negative event as above, you can practise changing your unhealthy negative emotions to their healthy equivalents by changing your specific unhealthy beliefs to specific healthy beliefs. REI is based on this principle.

What follows is a set of instructions for using both Ellis's and Maultsby's versions of REI. You will note that in both techniques you are encouraged to first respond to a negative situation with an unhealthy negative emotion, before changing this to a healthy negative emotion. This is realistic, since change frequently involves changing an unhealthy process to a healthy one totally eradicating the unhealthy process so that one only experiences the healthy one. Thus, both forms of REI have been devised to reflect a realistic view of the change process.

Instructions for using rational-emotive imagery: Ellis version

1 Take a situation in which you disturbed yourself and identify the aspect of the situation you were most disturbed about (i.e. the critical *A*).
2 Close your eyes and imagine the situation as vividly as possible and focus on the critical *A*.
3 Allow yourself to really experience the unhealthy negative emotion that you felt at the time while still focusing intently on the critical *A*. Ensure

that your unhealthy negative emotion is *one* of the following: anxiety, depression, shame, guilt, hurt, unhealthy anger, unhealthy jealousy, unhealthy envy.

4 Really experience this disturbed emotion for a moment or two and then change your emotional response to a healthy negative emotion. All the time focus intently on the critical *A* within the chosen situation. Do not change the intensity of the emotion, just the emotion. Thus, if your original unhealthy negative emotion was anxiety, change this to concern; if it was depression, change it to sadness. Change shame to disappointment, guilt to remorse, hurt to sorrow, unhealthy anger to healthy anger, unhealthy jealousy to healthy jealousy and unhealthy envy to healthy envy. Again change the unhealthy negative emotion to its healthy alternative but keep the level of intensity of the new emotion equivalent to the old emotion. Keep experiencing this new emotion for about five minutes, all the time focusing on the critical *A*. If you go back to the old, unhealthy negative emotion, bring the new healthy negative emotion back.
5 At the end of five minutes ask yourself how you changed your emotion.
6 Make sure that you changed your emotional response by changing your specific unhealthy belief to its healthy alternative. If you did not do so (if, for example, you changed your emotion by changing the critical *A* to make it less negative or neutral or by holding an indifference belief about the critical *A*) do the exercise again and keep doing this until you have changed your emotion only by changing your specific unhealthy belief to its healthy alternative.

If you experience trouble implementing the Ellis version of REI, it may be that you are facing one of the common difficulties that people encounter with this technique. Below is a list of such common problems with suggested remedies.

Problem You haven't chosen a specific negative situation.
Remedy Make sure that the situation you have chosen is specific enough to imagine.

Problem You think that unless you can imagine the situation vividly it is not worth using Ellis's REI.
Remedy Use Ellis's REI even though your image may not be vivid.

Problem You haven't selected the critical *A*.
Remedy Use Windy's magic question to identify the critical *A* (see p. 60).

Problem You have tried to change more than one unhealthy negative emotion.
Remedy Select the *one* unhealthy negative emotion that predominated in the emotional episode.

Problem You have been too vague in the choice of your target unhealthy negative emotion (e.g. 'I felt bad' or 'I felt upset').
Remedy Choose one *specific* unhealthy negative emotion from the following list: anxiety, depression, shame, guilt, hurt, unhealthy anger, unhealthy jealousy, unhealthy envy.

Problem You have chosen a *healthy* negative emotion to change.
Remedy Make sure that you have selected a situation in which you disturbed yourself. If so, select an unhealthy negative emotion to change. If not, select a situation in which you did disturb yourself.

Problem You changed your unhealthy negative emotion to another unhealthy negative emotion.
Remedy Select the alternative healthy negative emotion to the unhealthy negative emotion you have targeted and use the REI to change your emotion to this selected emotion.

Problem You successfully changed your unhealthy negative emotion to its healthy equivalent but you did so without changing your specific unhealthy belief to its healthy alternative.
Remedy Ensure that you achieved your emotional transformation only by changing your specific unhealthy belief to its alternative specific healthy belief.

Problem You changed your unhealthy negative emotion to a less intense healthy negative emotion. The problem with doing this is that you are also decreasing the importance of your specific healthy belief (e.g. you are reducing the importance of your full preference and reducing your rating of badness in your anti-awfulizing belief).
Remedy Ensure that the intensity of your healthy negative emotion is equivalent to the intensity of your unhealthy negative emotion.

Problem You stopped the exercise as soon as you correctly changed your unhealthy negative emotion to its healthy alternative.
Remedy Stay with your new healthy negative emotion (and the associated healthy belief) for the full five minutes so that you can benefit from the technique.

If, after you have implemented the above remedies, you still have difficulty with this technique, discuss it with your REBT therapist if you are consulting one. Alternatively try using the Maultsby version of REI (see below).

Figure 12.3 gives Oliver's account of how he used the Ellis version of REI. Note the error that he makes in step 5 and how he rectified that error in step 6.

REI: Ellis version

1. **Identify a specific situation in which you disturbed yourself.**

   I received a memo to see my boss at the end of the working day.

2. **Close your eyes and vividly imagine the situation and focus on the aspect of the situation that you were most disturbed about (i.e. the critical *A*).**

   I focused on the scenario that my boss was going to criticize my work.

3. **Allow yourself to really experience the unhealthy negative emotion that you felt at the time while still focusing intently on the critical *A*. Ensure that your unhealthy negative emotion is *one* of the following: anxiety, depression, shame, guilt, hurt, unhealthy anger, unhealthy jealousy, unhealthy envy.**

   I allowed myself to feel anxious about my boss's criticism.

4. **Really experience this disturbed emotion for a moment or two and then change your emotional response to a healthy negative emotion, all the time focusing intently on the critical *A* within the chosen situation. Do not change the intensity of the emotion, just the emotion. Thus, if your original unhealthy negative emotion was anxiety change this to concern; if it was depression change it to sadness. Change shame to disappointment, guilt to remorse, hurt to sorrow, unhealthy anger to healthy anger, unhealthy jealousy to healthy jealousy and unhealthy envy to healthy envy. Again change the unhealthy negative emotion to its healthy alternative but keep the level of intensity of the new emotion equivalent to the old emotion. Keep experiencing this new emotion for about five minutes, all the time focusing on the critical *A*. If you go back to the old, unhealthy negative emotion, bring the new healthy negative emotion back.**

   I changed my feelings of anxiety about being criticized by my boss to those of concern.

5. **At the end of five minutes ask yourself how you changed your emotion.**

   I changed my feelings by telling myself that while my boss will criticize me, he is generally pleased with my work.

6. **Make sure that you changed your emotional response by changing your specific unhealthy belief to its healthy alternative. If you did not do so (if, for example, you changed your emotion by changing the critical *A* to make it less negative or neutral or by holding an indifference belief about the critical *A*), do the exercise again and keep doing this until you have changed your emotion only by changing your specific unhealthy belief to its healthy alternative.**

   I recognized that I had changed my feelings of anxiety to concern by introducing a positive element into the critical A (i.e. that my boss is generally pleased with my work). As such I did not change my feelings by changing my beliefs. When I did the exercise again, I focused only on my boss's criticism and changed my feelings of anxiety to concern by changing my specific unhealthy belief 'My boss must not criticize my work and if he does it will prove that I am a stupid person' to its healthy alternative 'I don't want my boss to criticize my work but I am not immune from such criticism. His criticism would not make me a stupid person. It would prove that I am a fallible human being whose work may not have been good on that occasion'.

Figure 12.3 Oliver's account of his use of Ellis's version of rational-emotive imagery.

Use Figure 12.4 to reflect on your use of Ellis's REI so that you can correct any errors that you may have made.

The Maultsby version of REI differs from the Ellis version in one significant respect. In the Ellis version you gain practice at changing your unhealthy negative emotion (UNE) to an alternative healthy negative emotion (HNE) by changing your unhealthy beliefs to healthy beliefs *implicitly*. Thus you do not bring about emotional change by deliberately and explicitly rehearsing a specific healthy belief. Rather, you change your UNE to an HNE and then check that you did so by changing your unhealthy belief to its healthy alternative and you persist with the exercise until you are satisfied that you have brought about emotional change by belief change.

In the Maultsby version of REI, by contrast, you effect a change in your emotion (from unhealthy negative to healthy negative) by *deliberately* and *explicitly* changing your unhealthy belief to an alternative healthy belief as will be shown below.

Instructions for using rational-emotive imagery: Maultsby version

1 Identify a specific situation in which you disturbed yourself.
2 Close your eyes and vividly imagine the situation and focus on the aspect of the situation that you were most disturbed about (i.e. the critical *A*).
3 As you do so, rehearse your specific unhealthy belief about the critical *A* until you experience the *one* major unhealthy negative emotion that typified your disturbance, choose one from anxiety, depression, shame, guilt, hurt, unhealthy anger, unhealthy jealousy or unhealthy envy, and stay with this feeling for a moment or two.
4 While still imagining the same situation and focusing on the critical *A*, change your specific unhealthy belief to its healthy alternative and stay with this new belief until you experience a healthy negative emotion at the equivalent level of intensity to the unhealthy alternative. Your healthy negative emotion should be the direct alternative to the unhealthy negative emotion that you identified in step 3, and it will be one of the following: concern, sadness, disappointment, remorse, sorrow, healthy anger, healthy jealousy or healthy envy.
5 Stay with this specific healthy belief for about five minutes, all the time imagining the negative situation and focusing on the critical *A*. If you return to the former specific unhealthy belief, bring the new healthy belief back. If necessary, strongly repeat this healthy belief until you have made the emotional shift.

In checking your experiences of using Maultsby's version of REI refer to several of the points I covered when discussing troubleshooting problems in

REI: Ellis version

1. Identify a specific situation in which you disturbed yourself.

2. Close your eyes and vividly imagine the situation and focus on the aspect of the situation that you were most disturbed about (i.e. the critical *A*).

3. Allow yourself to really experience the unhealthy negative emotion that you felt at the time while still focusing intently on the critical *A*. Ensure that your unhealthy negative emotion is *one* of the following: anxiety, depression, shame, guilt, hurt, unhealthy anger, unhealthy jealousy, unhealthy envy.

4. Really experience this disturbed emotion for a moment or two and then change your emotional response to a healthy negative emotion, all the time focusing intently on the critical *A* within the chosen situation. Do not change the intensity of the emotion, just the emotion. Thus, if your original unhealthy negative emotion was anxiety change this to concern; if it was depression change it to sadness. Change shame to disappointment, guilt to remorse, hurt to sorrow, unhealthy anger to healthy anger, unhealthy jealousy to healthy jealousy and unhealthy envy to healthy envy. Again change the unhealthy negative emotion to its healthy alternative but keep the level of intensity of the new emotion equivalent to the old emotion. Keep experiencing this new emotion for about five minutes, all the time focusing on the critical *A*. If you go back to the old, unhealthy negative emotion, bring the new healthy negative emotion back.

5. At the end of five minutes ask yourself how you changed your emotion.

6. Make sure that you changed your emotional response by changing your specific unhealthy belief to its healthy alternative. If you did not do so (if, for example, you changed your emotion by changing the critical *A* to make it less negative or neutral or by holding an indifference belief about the critical *A*), do the exercise again and keep doing this until you have changed your emotion only by changing your specific unhealthy belief to its healthy alternative.

Figure 12.4 Your account of your use of Ellis's version of rational-emotive imagery.

using the Ellis version (see pp. 193–195). In particular, make sure that you brought about emotional change by rehearsing your specific healthy belief. If not, repeat the exercise until you do so.

Figure 12.5 gives Oliver's account of how he used the Maultsby version of REI.

Use Figure 12.6 to reflect on your use of Maultsby's REI so that you can correct any errors that you may have made.

While both versions of REI have been devised for use to strengthen your conviction in your specific healthy beliefs (and therefore you will be doing this while imagining specific negative events) you can also use REI to strengthen your conviction in your core healthy beliefs. What you do in this situation is:

- identify the core unhealthy belief that you wish to weaken and the corresponding core healthy belief that you wish to strengthen;
- list specific situations in which you hold the core unhealthy belief and identify the relevant critical *A* for each situation;
- finally, identify the specific healthy beliefs that would enable you to respond healthily to the critical *A* in each situation.

Use this information in either the Ellis version of REI or the Maultsby version. Don't forget that in both versions of REI you are asked to imagine specific situations. So work your way through a list of specific situations that you have compiled (see above).

My final point concerns how frequently you should practise REI. My suggestion is that you practise it several times a day and aim for 30 minutes daily practice (when you are not doing any other therapy homework). You might practise it more frequently and for a longer period of time when you are about to face a negative situation about which you are likely to disturb yourself. When you are doing other therapy homework 15 minutes daily REI practice will suffice.

Teaching healthy beliefs to others

Another way of strengthening your conviction in your healthy beliefs is to teach them to others. I am not suggesting that you play the role of therapist to friends and relatives nor am I suggesting that you foist these ideas on people who are not interested in discussing them. Rather, I am suggesting that you teach healthy beliefs to people who hold the alternative unhealthy beliefs and are interested in hearing what you have to say on the subject. When you do this, and in particular when the other person argues with your viewpoint in defending their position, you get the experience of responding to their arguments with persuasive arguments of your own. In doing so you strengthen your conviction in your own healthy beliefs. I suggest that you do this after you

REI: Maultsby version

1. **Identify a specific situation in which you disturbed yourself.**

   I received a memo to see my boss at the end of the working day.

2. **Close your eyes and vividly imagine the situation and focus on the aspect of the situation that you were most disturbed about (i.e. the critical *A*).**

   I focused on the scenario that my boss was going to criticize my work.

3. **As you do so, rehearse your specific unhealthy belief about the critical *A* until you experience the *one* major unhealthy negative emotion that typified your disturbance (choose one from anxiety, depression, shame, guilt, hurt, unhealthy anger, unhealthy jealousy or unhealthy envy) and stay with this feeling for a moment or two.**

   I rehearsed the following specific unhealthy belief until I began to feel anxious 'My boss must not criticize my work and if he does it proves that I am a stupid person'.

4. **While still imagining the same situation and focusing on the critical *A*, change your specific unhealthy belief to its healthy alternative and stay with this new belief until you experience a healthy negative emotion at the equivalent level of intensity to the unhealthy alternative. Your healthy negative emotion should be the direct alternative to the unhealthy negative emotion you identified in step 3 and will be one of the following: concern, sadness, disappointment, remorse, sorrow, healthy anger, healthy jealousy or healthy envy.**

   I changed my specific unhealthy belief to the following specific healthy belief until I felt concerned, but not anxious 'I don't want my boss to criticize my work but I am not immune from such criticism. His criticism would not make me a stupid person. It would prove that I am a fallible human being whose work may not have been good on that occasion'.

5. **Stay with this specific healthy belief for about five minutes all the time imagining the negative situation and focusing on the critical *A*. If you return to the former specific unhealthy belief, bring the new healthy belief back. If necessary, strongly repeat this healthy belief until you have made the emotional shift.**

   I struggled to keep to my healthy belief but did so after repeating it to myself very strongly.

Figure 12.5 Oliver's account of his use of Maultsby's version of rational-emotive imagery.

REI: Maultsby version

1. Identify a specific situation in which you disturbed yourself.

2. Close your eyes and vividly imagine the situation and focus on the aspect of the situation that you were most disturbed about (i.e. the critical *A*).

3. As you do so, rehearse your specific unhealthy belief about the critical *A* until you experience the *one* major unhealthy negative emotion that typified your disturbance (choose one from anxiety, depression, shame, guilt, hurt, unhealthy anger, unhealthy jealousy or unhealthy envy) and stay with this feeling for a moment or two.

4. While still imagining the same situation and focusing on the critical *A*, change your specific unhealthy belief to its healthy alternative and stay with this new belief until you experience a healthy negative emotion at the equivalent level of intensity to the unhealthy alternative. Your healthy negative emotion should be the direct alternative to the unhealthy negative emotion you identified in step 3 and will be one of the following: concern, sadness, disappointment, remorse, sorrow, healthy anger, healthy jealousy or healthy envy.

5. Stay with this specific healthy belief for about five minutes all the time imagining the negative situation and focusing on the critical *A*. If you return to the former specific unhealthy belief, bring the new healthy belief back. If necessary, strongly repeat this healthy belief until you have made the emotional shift.

Figure 12.6 Your account of your use of Maultsby's version of rational-emotive imagery.

have developed competence in using the written and tape-recorded versions of the zig-zag technique, since the back and forth discussion which often ensues when you attempt to teach healthy beliefs to others is reminiscent of the zig-zag method.

Other issues

In closing I want to point out that you can use some of the methods that I have discussed in earlier chapters to strengthen your conviction in your healthy beliefs. Thus, you can use the forceful self-statements discussed on pp. 133–134 in Chapter 8 to strengthen your conviction in both your specific and your core healthy beliefs. With reference to strengthening your specific healthy beliefs, you can use these forceful self-statements while facing relevant negative situations in actuality and in imagery. Thus, if your specific healthy belief is 'I want to be approved by my friend Bill but it isn't essential for him to approve of me. I can accept myself whether Bill approves of me or not', you can repeat this to yourself forcefully while actually facing Bill at a time when it is likely that he will disapprove of you or while imagining Bill disapproving of you.

With reference to strengthening your core healthy beliefs, you can rehearse these to yourself at various times while thinking of classes of negative situations that reflect the theme of your healthy belief. For example, if your core healthy belief is 'I want to be approved by my friends but they don't have to approve of me. I can accept myself whether they approve of me or not', you can repeat this to yourself in a forceful way while thinking broadly about your friends not approving of you.

As I have mentioned before (and in particular in Chapter 8), perhaps the most powerful way of strengthening one of your healthy beliefs is to rehearse it and act on it while thinking in realistic ways that are consistent with it. When all these systems are working together in synchrony and you keep them in synchrony repeatedly, you maximize your chances of strengthening your conviction in your healthy beliefs.

Chapter 13

Goal achievement and beyond

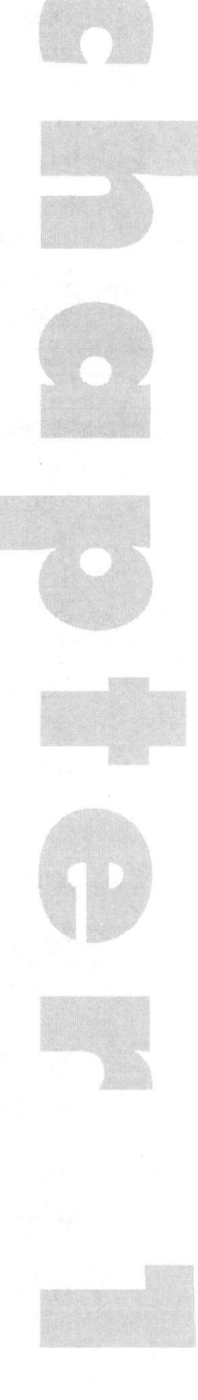

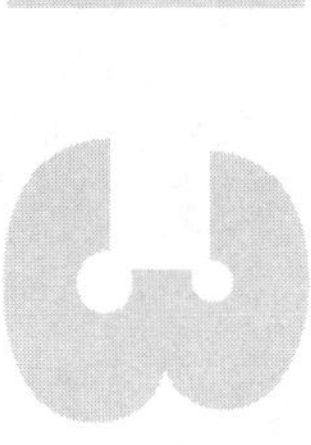

We have now come to the final chapter in this REBT workbook. Here I will consider how you can evaluate the outcome of the work you have done on yourself and how you can maintain your therapeutic gains.

Evaluating outcome

If you have regularly practised the skills that I have taught you in this book then the time has come to evaluate the fruits of your labours. There are several ways to do this.

Have you achieved your goals?

You will recall that in Chapter 3 I encouraged you to set two types of goals:

1 overcoming psychological problem (OPP) goals;
2 personal development (PD) goals.

I made the important point that, most often, you need to have made reasonable progress at achieving your OPP goals first before you can begin to make progress at achieving your PD goals.

Evaluating overcoming psychological problem goals

When you come to evaluate your OPP goals I suggest that you ask yourself the following questions:

1 Have I achieved this goal?
2 If so, how can I capitalize on it?
3 If not, what do I need to do to achieve it?
4 How might I stop myself from doing what I need to do to achieve my goal?
5 What can I do to overcome these obstacles?

Here is an example of how Freda, one of the people who has used this workbook, answered these questions in relation to the following OPP goal.

> *When I see my friends with their babies and I focus on the fact that I don't have what they have, my goal is to experience healthy envy rather than unhealthy envy and to remind myself of what I do have in my life as well as what I don't have, rather than drinking to blot out my feelings.*

1 HAVE I ACHIEVED THIS GOAL?

I have made a lot of progress towards achieving this goal, but there are times when I still feel unhealthily envious. However, I no longer drink to blot out my feelings. I generally remind myself of what I have in life, but occasionally I forget to do this.

2 IF SO, HOW CAN I CAPITALIZE ON IT?

Not applicable.

3 IF NOT, WHAT DO I NEED TO DO TO ACHIEVE IT?

I need to practise reviewing my healthy belief 'I'd like to have children but it isn't absolutely necessary that I have them. It's sad that others have what I don't have but this isn't, repeat isn't, the end of the world' when I'm with Lucy and Jane, with whom I feel unhealthy envy these days.

4 HOW MIGHT I STOP MYSELF FROM DOING WHAT I NEED TO DO TO ACHIEVE MY GOAL?

I might get caught up with the strong feelings of unhealthy envy and forget to challenge my unhealthy belief.

5 WHAT CAN I DO TO OVERCOME THESE OBSTACLES?

I can write my healthy belief on 3 × 5 card and consult it when I'm about to meet Lucy or Jane. I can also practise Ellis's version of REI on a daily basis instead of twice a week.

Once you have answered these questions, if applicable, it is important that you follow through on the course of action that you have suggested to overcome such obstacles.

Evaluating personal development goals

After you have made good strides at achieving your OPP goal, you can begin to turn your attention to your personal development (PD) goal on each issue. As I discussed in Chapter 3, your PD goal is often more speculative than your

OPP goal in that you don't know that you will achieve it even if you put in the effort. I made the point in Chapter 3 that when I had achieved my OPP goal of being concerned rather than anxious about public speaking, I turned my attention to my PD goal of enjoying talking in public. I knew that my anxiety would interfere with any enjoyment I would derive from public speaking, but I did not know whether I would enjoy it once I was largely over my anxiety. The only way I could judge whether or not I could achieve my PD goal was to speak up in public as often as practicable, learn from my experience and decide whether I needed some additional skills to aid my quest to enjoy public speaking.

Thus, if you are to achieve your PD goals you need to do three things:

1 persist
2 be willing to learn from your experience and to change your behaviour if needed
3 acquire new skills if necessary.

If you do all three things, you may not be successful at achieving your PD goal but you will have done all you could to reach this goal. Consequently, you may have to conclude that the goal is, for one reason or another, not for you.

When you come to evaluate your PD goals I suggest that you ask yourself the following questions:

1 Have I achieved this goal?
2 If so, how can I capitalize on this?
3 If not, what do I need to do to achieve it? In particular do I need to learn new skills? Are there any other issues that I need to consider?
4 How might I stop myself from doing what I need to do to achieve my PD goal? In particular have I relapsed on my OPP goal and am I continuing to disturb myself on this issue? Have I been persistent in my behaviour?
5 What can I do to overcome these obstacles?

Once Freda had achieved her OPP goal, she worked at achieving the following PD goal.

To enjoy being with friends when they have their babies with them.

After she had worked to achieve this goal for a significant period of time, Freda answered the following questions in relation to her PD goal.

1 HAVE I ACHIEVED THIS GOAL?

No.

2 IF SO, HOW CAN I CAPITALIZE ON THIS?

Not applicable.

3 IF NOT, WHAT DO I NEED TO DO TO ACHIEVE IT? IN PARTICULAR DO I NEED TO LEARN NEW SKILLS? ARE THERE ANY OTHER ISSUES THAT I NEED TO CONSIDER?

That is difficult to say. I have spent a lot of time with my friends and their babies. I've read books on babies and I've even been on a short child-development course. I reluctantly conclude that I don't enjoy being with my friends when they have their babies with them and that my PD goal is probably not achievable at the moment. I don't think that I need to learn new skills. I am good with babies. I don't think that there are other issues that I need to consider.

4 HOW MIGHT I STOP MYSELF FROM DOING WHAT I NEED TO DO TO ACHIEVE MY PD GOAL? IN PARTICULAR HAVE I RELAPSED ON MY OPP GOAL AND AM I CONTINUING TO DISTURB MYSELF ON THIS ISSUE? HAVE I BEEN PERSISTENT IN MY BEHAVIOUR?

I really think that I have done all I can to enjoy this experience. I have persisted in meeting with friends. I can also honestly say that I don't feel unhealthily envious about not having children. Indeed, the more time I spend with my friends' babies, the more relieved I feel that I don't have children. I have really surprised myself about this.

5 WHAT CAN I DO TO OVERCOME THESE OBSTACLES?

Not applicable.

Once you have answered these questions, if applicable, it is important that you follow through on the course of action that you have suggested to overcome such obstacles.

Have you changed your core beliefs?

A second way to evaluate the outcome of your efforts is to ask yourself whether or not you have changed your core beliefs. In particular have you weakened your conviction in your core unhealthy beliefs and strengthened your conviction in your core healthy beliefs? If so, the following will be true.

1 You will experience healthy negative emotions when you face situations with a theme central to your core belief. If you do experience unhealthy negative emotions under these conditions, you will quickly use this as a cue to rehearse your core healthy belief (or a specific variant of it) and will soon return to your healthy emotion.
2 You will act in ways that are consistent with your core healthy belief when you face such situations. This behaviour will be constructive and you will resist any urge that you experience to go back to previous unconstructive behaviour. If you do return to such behaviour, you will intervene quickly by rehearsing your core healthy belief (or a specific variant of it) and go back to acting constructively.
3 The inferences that you make about such situations and about other related matters will be balanced and realistic rather than skewed and distorted. If you do make distorted inferences you will quickly realize this and correct them.

Let's suppose that you have been working on changing a core unhealthy belief and want to evaluate the extent to which you believe its healthy alternative. How can you do this? I suggest that you do the following.

1 Write down the core unhealthy belief that you have been working to change.
2 Write down the core alternative healthy belief.
3 Note the theme of the core unhealthy/healthy belief.
4 When you encounter situations which reflect the above theme are you still experiencing unhealthy negative emotions in the face of certain 'theme' situations? If so, list those situations and your unhealthy emotional responses and take steps to deal with them more productively so that you can respond to the situations with healthy negative emotions. In particular focus on the people involved if this is relevant.
5 If you are reacting to certain 'theme' situations with unconstructive behaviour, list those situations and your unhealthy behavioural responses and take steps to deal with them more productively so that you can respond to the situations with constructive behaviour. Again focus on the people involved if this is relevant.
6 Ask yourself whether or not you are still overestimating the extent to which your theme will be present in situations as judged by neutral observers. If so, list the situations where you do this and take remedial steps.
7 Ask yourself whether or not your subsequent thinking in theme-based

situations is unrealistic as judged by neutral observers. If so, list the situations where you do this and take remedial steps.

8 Are you avoiding theme-based situations when it is not in your best interests to do so? If so, list these situations and take remedial steps.

Here is how one of my clients responded to these points.

1 Write down the core unhealthy belief that you have been working to change.
I must be approved by significant others. If I'm not it proves that I am an unlikeable person.

2 Write down the core alternative healthy belief.
I want to be approved by significant others but it's not essential that I receive such approval. I am not an unlikeable person. I am a fallible person who can be approved of and disapproved of.

3 Note the theme of the core unhealthy/healthy belief.
Lack of approval.

4 When you encounter situations that reflect the above theme, do you still experience unhealthy negative emotions in the face of certain 'theme' situations? If so, list those situations and your unhealthy emotional responses and take steps to deal with them more productively so that you can respond to the situations with healthy negative emotions. In particular focus on the people involved if this is relevant.
I still feel anxious when I am in the company of the president of the company, especially when I have to interact with him in informal situations. To deal with this I will practise the Ellis version of REI daily and then I will undertake to speak to him at every informal situation instead of trying to avoid him. In doing so I will rehearse the relevant specific variant of my core healthy belief. In all other situations where I may not be approved, I tend to feel concerned rather than anxious.

5 If you are reacting to certain 'theme' situations with unconstructive behaviour, list those situations and your unhealthy behavioural responses and take steps to deal with the situations more productively so that you can respond to them with constructive behaviour. Again focus on the people involved if this is relevant.
As I have said, I tend to avoid speaking to the company president at informal gatherings. So I will undertake to talk to him at informal gatherings while rehearsing my healthy belief.

6 Ask yourself whether or not you are still overestimating the extent to

which your theme will be present in situations as judged by neutral observers. If so, list the situations where you do this and take remedial steps.
I still tend to anticipate not being approved of by people in authority even though in most cases, I don't disturb myself about this lack of approval. I need to rehearse my healthy belief before encountering such authority figures and then look objectively at the possibility that they will not approve of me.

7 Ask yourself whether or not your subsequent thinking in theme-based situations is unrealistic as judged by neutral observers. If so, list the situations where you do this and take remedial steps.
I still tend to think that if I am not approved of at work then I will lose my job despite the fact that I have consistently received good reports by my immediate boss. I will challenge my need for approval and show myself that lack of approval isn't awful and that there is little evidence that I will lose my job if I do not receive approval from people at work.

8 Are you avoiding theme-based situations when it is not in your best interests to do so? If so, list these situations and take remedial steps.
See my answer to points 4 and 5 above.

Relapse prevention and ongoing psychological maintenance

Once you have achieved your goals and made significant progress at strengthening your conviction in your core healthy beliefs, you might think that you can rest on your laurels and that maintaining psychological health will be a breeze. If you think this you are sadly mistaken. There are two reasons why you cannot rest on your psychological laurels:

1 as a human you have a tendency to backslide and suffer lapses in your progress;
2 maintaining psychological health requires work.

To do proper justice to these two issues would require an entire book so what I will do here is to give you some important suggestions on how to prevent a relapse and how to maintain your therapeutic gains.

Relapse prevention

In this section I will make some suggestions on how to prevent a relapse. I make an important distinction between a 'lapse' and a 'relapse'. I define a lapse as 'a partial return to a problem state' and a relapse as 'a full return to a problem state'. In order to prevent a relapse I suggest that you do the following:

1 ACCEPT THAT LAPSES IN YOUR PROGRESS WILL OCCUR WITHOUT LIKING THIS FACT

Once you have achieved your OPP goals it would be nice to think that you could never lose these gains, but sadly this is not the case. In the same way that progress towards your goals is uneven and can take the form of two steps forward and one back, and sometimes one step forward and two back, the same is the case when you have achieved your goals. There are three major reasons why lapses in your progress will in all probability occur:

- change by its nature is rarely, if ever, linear and has an up and down quality to it;
- you may stop working to maintain your progress, believing wrongly that you do not need to because you hold an an irrational belief based on low frustration tolerance about maintenance work;
- you are ill-equipped to deal with certain events and when you encounter them you disturb yourself.

Consequently, an important attitude for you to cultivate in relation to lapses is to accept that they will in all probability occur, without liking this grim fact. If you find yourself disturbing yourself about the prospect or the reality of experiencing a lapse, then use this as an opportunity to practise the skills that you have learned in this workbook to overcome your disturbance. This will enable you to take the next step.

2 DEAL WITH THE LAPSE AS SOON AS YOU NOTICE IT

The best way to deal with a lapse is to deal with it as soon as you notice it. This involves you guarding against the very human tendency of hoping that if you ignore something it will go away. Going against this 'ostrich-like' behaviour will help you to deal effectively with the lapse as soon as it is practicable for you to do so. In doing so you can utilize your own devised shortened form of the DRF-2 or, if you are sufficiently advanced in the use of the skills outlined in this workbook, you can ask yourself questions such as 'What am I demanding in this situation?' and challenge the identified irrational or composite unhealthy belief. The goal of both approaches is for you to rehearse the resultant rational or composite healthy belief while acting and thinking in ways that are consistent with it.

3 IDENTIFY AND DEAL WITH YOUR VULNERABILITY FACTORS

Another important strand in relapse prevention requires you to identify factors that render you vulnerable to relapse and tackling such factors in a systematic and sensible way. The following can be vulnerability factors.

Theme-based situations about which you are likely to disturb yourself where specific people are involved

After he had reached his OPP goal Oliver thought he was particularly vulnerable to facing the head of his corporation when there was a chance of that person criticizing his work in front of other people. This situation contained the theme 'criticism' and the particular person that Oliver felt particularly vulnerable to 'the head of the corporation in which he worked'. Putting these two aspects together we have the context in which Oliver was vulnerable to disturbing himself, i.e. 'facing the head of my corporation when there is a chance of that person criticizing my work in front of other people'.

Once you have identified these theme-based/significant other vulnerability factors it is important that you practise facing such situations while rehearsing your healthy belief and acting and thinking in ways that are consistent with this healthy belief. This can be done in your mind's eye using rational-emotive imagery (see Chapter 12) and in real-life settings using the hierarchy method described in Chapter 8 if there are a number of such situational factors. If facing such factors is not realistic (e.g. Oliver might suffer real penalties if he deliberately exposed shoddy work to the head of his corporation), you can use REI as an alternative to real-life practice and as a way of preparing yourself to face a situation in which your critical *A* happens even though you have done nothing to bring it about. Thus, Oliver could practise REI before group meetings with the head of his corporation in which he may receive criticism from the corporation head even though he will do nothing to court such criticism.

If, on the other hand, facing such factors is realistic you can use REI as a way of mentally rehearsing your healthy belief in the face of the imagined critical *A* before actually facing that *A* in real life.

List your theme-based/significant other vulnerability factors in Figure 13.1 and deal with them as suggested.

Figure 13.2 shows how one person completed this form.

Lifestyle factors

There are a host of lifestyle factors that can serve as vulnerability factors in the sense that they increase the chances that you will disturb yourself about

Theme-based/significant other vulnerability factors	How I can deal with these factors
1	1
2	2
3	3
4	4
5	5

Figure 13.1 Identifying and dealing with theme-based/significant other vulnerability factors.

Theme-based/significant other vulnerability factors	How I can deal with these factors
1. Being with my drinking friends and them calling me a wimp for drinking orange juice	1. a) Practise rational-emotive imagery and rehearse my self-acceptance belief in the face of my friends calling me a wimp b) Practise asserting myself when they call me a wimp c) If things get really rough, I will leave the situation rather than drink
2. Feeling lonely and seeing people drinking and enjoying themselves on television	2. a) Challenge the belief that while I may want to be with people right now, I don't need to be with them b) Remind myself that I am watching television and that if I were to drink, any enjoyment I will experience which I do not need to have will soon give way to my addictive behaviour c) After I have challenged my healthy beliefs about not being with people and about having a drink, I will seek out company because I want company not because I need it d) Find a vital absorbing interest which I can pursue on my own
3. Being let down by a close friend	3. a) Challenge the belief that my friend absolutely should not have let me down b) Tell my friend how I felt about his behaviour and try to repair my relationship with that person

Figure 13.2 Identifying and dealing with theme-based/significant other vulnerability factors – an example.

situations that you might otherwise not disturb yourself about if these factors were absent. The following is a list of common lifestyle factors which may render you more vulnerable to lapses in your psychological problems:

- lack of sleep
- lack of exercise
- use of addictive and recreational drugs
- alcohol abuse.

The greater the number of these lifestyle factors you have in your life the harder you will find it to maintain your psychological equilibrium and the more you will tend to experience lapses and relapses in your problems. This is leaving aside the damage that these lifestyle factors have on your physical health. If you sleep well, carry out a sensible exercise regime, refrain from taking addictive and recreational drugs and do not abuse alcohol then you will help to ensure that you are in the best condition to deal with the psychological vulnerability factors discussed in the previous section.

So, if you have one or more of the above lifestyle factors discuss them with your REBT therapist who will point you in the right direction for help, or if you are using this workbook on your own consult your GP in the first instance who will do the same.

4 DON'T DISTURB YOURSELF ABOUT THE PROSPECT OF A RELAPSE

Strangely enough, one way of hastening a relapse is to disturb yourself about the prospect of experiencing one. When you disturb yourself about the prospect of having a relapse several things happen.

1 You make yourself anxious and are thus less likely to deal constructively with your theme-based vulnerability factors than you would do if you were concerned, but not anxious, about a relapse.
2 In your mind you overestimate the chances of a relapse happening with the consequence that you spend more time being preoccupied with this than you do in taking constructive steps to prevent such a relapse.
3 You underestimate your ability to cope with a relapse and once again this has the effect of you not taking the necessary steps to deal with lapses, thus rendering you more vulnerable to relapse.

Consequently, it is important that you work on undisturbing yourself about the prospect of experiencing a relapse so that you are healthily concerned about this possibility rather than unhealthily anxious about it. You can do this by using the techniques that I have already taught you in this book. In particular, you may wish to use your own version of the DRF-2, or the full version as found in Appendix 1.

What should you do if you have followed all these steps and have still relapsed? I suggest that you use the skills that you have learned in this book to do the following.

1 Identify and deal with any disturbed feelings that you have about your relapse.
2 Work towards your OPP goal on the issue on which you relapsed. You will probably do this by using the same methods that helped you to achieve your goal before.

Once you have achieved your goal you are ready to learn from this experience of relapse. Do so by following the next steps.

1 Identify the point at which you began to lapse.
2 Identify and deal with the factors that were associated with this lapse. Check whether or not this course of action would have helped you to deal with this lapse and to ward off the relapse. If so move on to the next step. If not, discuss this issue with your REBT therapist or consult one for a time-limited consultation if you are using this workbook on your own (see Appendix 3).
3 Ask yourself how you stopped yourself from identifying and dealing with the lapse at the time. In particular, focus on the unhealthy beliefs that were at the core of your *in*action. Work to change these unhealthy beliefs and imagine yourself dealing with your lapse while rehearsing your healthy beliefs (perhaps using REI, see Chapter 12).
4 Make a careful note of signs that might indicate that you are experiencing a lapse again. Resolve to take effective action as soon as you identify these signs. Challenge and change any unhealthy beliefs that might impede you from taking such action.
5 Take effective action and note the results. If they are successful be pleased with your efforts and resolve to take such action in the future if needed. If your efforts are not successful, identify and deal with factors that you may not have considered earlier in the process. You may need the help of an REBT therapist if you get stuck on this point.

Maintaining psychological gains

You have now reached the final section of this workbook. I want to leave you on an optimistic, but realistic note. The optimistic note is that it is possible for you to maintain your psychological gains, the realistic note is that such maintenance requires ongoing work, not as much work as it takes to overcome your psychological problems in the first place but work none the less. If you accept the following points then you will be more likely to do such ongoing work.

1 Accept that as a human you have a natural tendency to drift back to old patterns of unhealthy thinking and behaviour if you don't work to maintain new patterns of healthy thinking and behaviour.
2 Accept that maintaining psychological health requires work in the same way as physical health does. You would not say for example 'my teeth are clean so I will never clean them again or I will only clean them when they hurt'. You clean them to maintain dental health. You recognize that the same principle applies to the arena of psychological health.

So what do I recommend? I suggest that you do the following:

1 Do a little to help yourself every day. Twenty minutes psychological workout using the skills I have taught you in this book should suffice. Choose the techniques that work best for you.
2 Concentrate on dealing with your vulnerability factors until they are no longer vulnerability factors. If you do this you will minimize (but not eradicate) your tendency to lapse. The best way to do this is to face these factors in reality while rehearsing your healthy beliefs before, during and after such encounters.
3 Identify areas which give you meaning in life and actively pursue them. Active engagement in such pursuits is better than passive engagement.

I could say a lot more about this latter point and related issues of how to move towards self-actualization but this warrants a book on its own (which I will write if this one is successful!). In the meantime you might want to read Chapters 6–10 of my book *Ten Steps to Positive Living* (Dryden 1994) if you wish to pursue your interest in this area.

You have now reached the end of this workbook. I appreciate your patience in staying with me and hope that you have derived benefit from the skills that I have taught you and that you have (hopefully) actively practised. I would very much like to learn of your experiences in using this workbook so that I can improve it in future editions. Please write to me c/o the publisher.

Thank you!

Appendix 1

Blank Dryden REBT form (DRF-2)

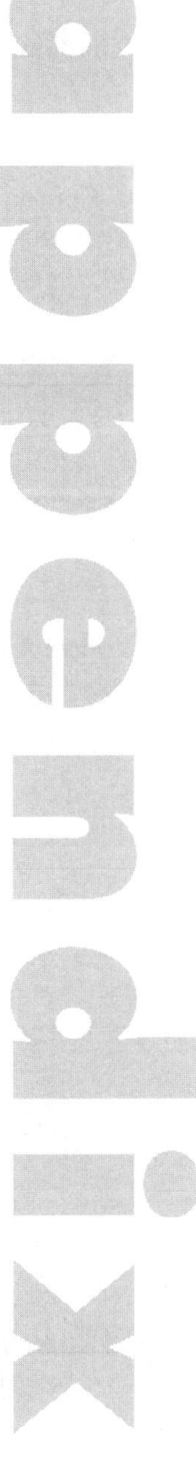

The Dryden REBT form (DRF-2)

1. **Situation:** briefly describe a specific situation in which you disturbed yourself

2. **C (Consequences):** Identify your major unhealthy negative emotion in this episode, choose one from: anxiety, depression, shame, guilt, hurt, unhealthy anger, unhealthy jealousy and unhealthy envy. Also specify how you acted (or 'felt like' acting) in this situation.

i) Emotional consequences =

ii) Behavioural consequences =

3. **Critical A (Activating event):** identify the aspect of the situation that you were most disturbed about at *C*.

4. **B (Beliefs):** identify your irrational beliefs about *A* and list their rational alternatives

i) **Demand =**	i) **Full preference =**
ii) **Awfulizing belief =**	ii) **Anti-awfulizing belief =**
iii) **Low frustration tolerance belief =**	iii **High frustration tolerance belief =**
iv) **Depreciation belief =**	iv) **Acceptance belief =**

5. **Select your demand** and the one other **irrational belief** (from the remaining three) that was at the core of your emotional and/or behavioural reaction to *A*. Also **select your full preference** and the **appropriate rational belief** and write down both sets of beliefs (which you can refer to as unhealthy and healthy beliefs respectively) side by side in the space below

Demand and irrational belief	**Full preference and rational belief**
(Unhealthy belief)	(Healthy belief)

6. **Emotional and behavioural goals**: identify what you would have preferred your healthy negative *emotion* to have been if you had responded constructively to *A*. Choose one from concern, sadness, disappointment, remorse, sorrow, healthy anger, healthy jealousy and healthy envy. Also specify how you would have preferred to have acted (or 'felt like' acting) if you had responded constructively to *A*

   i) Emotional goal =

   ii) Behavioural goal =

7. **Belief goal**: which belief listed in step 5 would help you to achieve your emotional and behavioural goals listed above?

8. **List persuasive arguments** that would help you to strengthen your conviction in the belief you listed in step 7 above and weaken your conviction in the other belief (see step 5)

   i)

   ii)

iii)

iv)

v)

vi)

vii)

viii)

ix)

9. **Deal with your doubts, reservations and objections**

Doubts about adopting my healthy belief:

and/or giving up my unhealthy belief:

Doubt, reservation, objection:

Response:

Doubt, reservation, objection:

Response:

Doubt, reservation, objection:

Response:

Doubt, reservation, objection:

Response:

Doubts about adopting my healthy emotion:

and/or giving up my unhealthy emotion:

Doubt, reservation, objection:

Response:

Doubt, reservation, objection:

Response:

Doubts about adopting my constructive behaviour:

and/or giving up my unconstructive behaviour:

Doubt, reservation, objection:

Response:

Doubt, reservation, objection:

Response:

10. List **homework assignments** that you can do to strengthen your conviction in your healthy belief and weaken your conviction in your unhealthy belief. Be specific concerning what you will do for homework, when you will do it and where you will do it. The best homework assignments enable you to rehearse your healthy belief while acting in ways that are consistent with it

    i)

    ii)

    iii)

    iv)

    v)

11. **Reconsider the critical A**: write down the situation that you listed in step 1 and the critical *A* listed in step 3. Then ask yourself whether or not the critical *A* is the best way of viewing the situation given all the evidence to hand (illustrative questions provided)

Situation:

Critical *A*:

Illustrative questions:

- How likely is it that the critical *A* happened (or might happen)?
- Would an objective jury agree that the critical *A* actually happened or might happen? If not, what would the jury's verdict be?
- Did I view (am I viewing) the situation realistically? If not, how could I have viewed (can I view) it more realistically?
- If I asked someone whom I could trust to give me an objective opinion about the truth or falsity of my inference about the situation at hand, what would the person say to me and why? How would this person encourage me to view the situation instead?
- If a friend had told me that they had faced (were facing or were about to face) the same situation as I faced and had made the same inference, what would I say to him/her about the validity of their inference and why? How would I encourage the person to view the situation instead?

Conclusion:

Appendix 2

A completed Dryden REBT form (DRF-2): Oliver's example

The Dryden REBT form (DRF-2)

1. **Situation:** briefly describe a specific situation in which you disturbed yourself
I received a memo to see my boss at the end of the working day.

2. ***C* (Consequences):** identify your major unhealthy negative emotion in this episode, choose one from: anxiety, depression, shame, guilt, hurt, unhealthy anger, unhealthy jealousy and unhealthy envy. Also specify how you acted (or 'felt like' acting) in this situation

   i) Emotional consequences = *Anxiety.*

   ii) Behavioural consequences = *I 'felt like' running away.*

3. **Critical *A* (Activating event):** identify the aspect of the situation that you were most disturbed about at *C*
My boss will criticize my work.

4. ***B* (Beliefs):** identify your irrational beliefs about *A* and list their rational alternatives

   i) **Demand** =
   My boss must not criticize my work.

   i) **Full preference** =
   I don't want my boss to criticize my work, but I'm not immune from such criticism.

   ii) **Awfulizing belief** =
   It would truly be awful if my boss criticized my work.

   ii) **Anti-awfulizing belief** =
   If my boss criticized my work, it would be bad but certainly not awful.

   iii) **Low frustration tolerance belief** =
   I couldn't bear it if my boss criticized my work.

   iii) **High frustration tolerance belief** =
   It would be hard for me to bear if my boss criticized my work but I could bear it and it would be worth bearing because it would help me to overcome my oversensitivity to criticism.

   iv) **Depreciation belief** =
   If my boss criticized my work, it would prove that I was a stupid person.

   iv) **Acceptance belief** =
   If my boss criticized my work it would not prove that I was a stupid person. It would prove that I was a fallible human being whose work may not have been good enough on that occasion.

5. ***Select your demand*** and the one other **irrational belief** that was at the core of your emotional and/or behavioural reaction to A. Also **select your full preference** and the **appropriate rational belief** and write down both sets of beliefs (which you can refer to as unhealthy and healthy beliefs respectively) side by side in the space below

Demand and irrational belief (Unhealthy belief)	**Full preference and rational belief** (Healthy belief)
My boss must not criticize my work and if he does it would prove that I was a stupid person.	*I don't want my boss to criticize my work but I am not immune from such criticism. His criticism would not make me a stupid person. It would prove that I was a fallible human whose work may not have been good enough on that occasion.*

6. **Emotional and behavioural goals:** identify what you would have preferred your healthy negative emotion to have been if you had responded constructively to A. Choose one from concern, sadness, remorse, disappointment, sorrow, healthy anger, healthy jealousy and healthy envy. Also specify how you would have preferred to have acted (or 'felt like' acting) if you had responded constructively to A

   i) Emotional goal = *Concern.*

   ii) Behavioural goal = *I would 'feel like' attending the meeting with my boss to face the music if he wants to criticize my work.*

7. **Belief goal:** which belief listed in step 5 would help you to achieve your emotional and behavioural goals listed above?

   I don't want my boss to criticize my work, but I am not immune from such criticism. His criticism would not make me a stupid person. It would prove that I was a fallible human being whose work may not have been good enough on that occasion.

8. **List persuasive arguments** that would help you to strengthen your conviction in the belief you listed in step 7 above and weaken your conviction in the other belief (see step 5)

   i) *It would be nice if I were immune from criticism from my boss, but I'm not. It is possible for him to criticize me and I'll have to get used to the idea without liking it.*
   ii) *While I don't want him to criticize me, it doesn't make sense for me to demand that he must not do so. To prefer him not to is flexible, while to demand it is rigid and you can't logically derive something rigid from something flexible.*
   iii) *As long as I demand that he mustn't criticize me and think I'm stupid if he does, then I'll be anxious about meeting him which won't help me to get on in the company or to focus on doing a good job in my work.*

iv) *Wanting my boss, on the other hand, not to criticize me without demanding that he mustn't do so will lead me to be healthily concerned and keep me on my toes in a positive way at work.*

v) *I can prove that I am not a stupid person if my boss criticizes me. His criticism is one act and being stupid would be my essence. One criticism hardly defines my essence.*

vi) *Conversely, I can prove that I am a fallible human being if my boss criticizes me. I am fallible whether he criticizes me or not. So my identity does not change if he criticizes me. By saying that his criticism makes me a stupid person I am implying that my identity is changed by his criticism.*

vii) *Even if I acted stupidly at work and my boss is correct to criticize me for my shoddy work, it still does not follow logically that I am a stupid person as a result. For me to conclude this is what philosophers would call a 'part–whole error', the illogical error of defining the whole of something on the basis of a part of it.*

9. Deal with your doubts, reservations and objections

Doubts about adopting my healthy belief: *I don't want my boss to criticize my work, but I am not immune from such criticism. His criticism would not make me a stupid person. It would prove that I was a fallible human being whose work wasn't that good on this occasion.*
and/or giving up my unhealthy belief: *My boss must not criticize my work, if he does it would prove that I was a stupid person.*

*Doubt, reservation, objection: *But surely people who do stupid things are stupid people.*

Response: *No they're not. They are people who have the capacity to do stupid things as well as non-stupid things. Just like me.*

*Doubt, reservation, objection: *But if I'm paid to do well at work, then I must do so. If I give up my 'must', I won't be motivated to do well.*

Response: *I'm paid to do the best I can at work. Being human means that I will act stupidly at times. If I do so too many times then I'll be fired. None of which proves that there is a law of nature decreeing that I must do well at work. I'll certainly strive to do so but I'm not a robot. My fallibility can't be programmed out of me. Also my full preference to do well will motivate me without the anxiety that goes with my demand.*

*Doubt, reservation, objection: *But I'm using being fallible as a cop-out, as an argument to excuse my shoddy work.*

Response: *No I'm not. If I have done shoddy work and I'm criticized for it I will take responsibility for my behaviour without regarding myself as stupid. Self-acceptance allows me to do both without copping-out.*

Doubts about adopting my healthy emotion: *Concern.*
and/or giving up my unhealthy emotion: *Anxiety.*

*Doubt, reservation, objection: *Being concerned about being criticized by my boss might lead me to be complacent at work. My anxiety will ensure that I'm not complacent.*

Response: *Having a 'don't care' attitude will lead to complacency but concern won't. Concern is based on my healthy belief which states that I prefer not to be criticized by my boss. This is not being complacent. It will motivate me to do well at work. My anxiety won't lead me to be complacent but it will impair my performance in a way that concern won't.*

Doubts about adopting my constructive behaviour: *'Feeling like' attending the meeting with my boss to face the music if he wants to criticize my work.*
and/or giving up my unconstructive behaviour: *'Feeling like' running away.*

*Doubt, reservation, objection: *Running away allows me to avoid the pain of being criticized. If I face the music I'll give myself more pain.*

Response: *Running away only serves to maintain my problem because it doesn't allow me to face the music while practising my healthy belief. It may give me short-term relief but it won't help me to overcome my anxiety about being criticized in the longer term.*

10. List **homework assignments** that you can do to strengthen your conviction in your healthy belief and weaken your conviction in your unhealthy belief. Be specific concerning what you will do for homework, when you will do it and where you will do it. The best homework assignments enable you to rehearse your healthy belief while acting in ways which are consistent with it

i) *To start with I'll ask my boss for feedback on work that I think I've done well. I'll do this on Wednesday and Friday at 4 pm after his tea break. In doing so I'll rehearse the belief that I'm not shoddy even if my work is. Rather, I'm a fallible human being who can work more effectively as well as ineffectively.*
ii) *Then if that goes well I'll do the same with work that I'm not so confident about the week after, also at the same time while rehearsing the same healthy belief.*
iii) *Then I'll discuss some work ideas that I'm not too confident about with some work colleagues during our morning coffee break. Before and during this I'll show myself that I can accept myself as a fallible human being capable of good and bad work even if they think I'm stupid for coming up with poor work ideas.*
iv) *If all that goes to plan, I'll extend my learning to the social area. I'll express myself with people that I've just met at a party and practise accepting myself if they criticize my social behaviour. I'll also show myself that while it is nice to be approved, I don't need these people's approval.*

11. Reconsider the critical *A*: write down the situation that you listed in step 1 and the critical *A* listed in step 3. Then ask yourself whether or not the critical *A* is the best way of viewing the situation given all the evidence to hand (illustrative questions provided)

Situation: *I received a memo to see my boss at the end of the working day*

Critical *A*: *My boss will criticize my work.*

Illustrative questions:

- How likely is it that the critical *A* happened (or might happen)?
- Would an objective jury agree that the critical *A* actually happened or might happen? If not, what would the jury's verdict be?
- Did I view (am I viewing) the situation realistically? If not, how could I have viewed (can I view) it more realistically?
- If I asked someone whom I could trust to give me an objective opinion about the truth or falsity of my inference about the situation at hand, what would the person say to me and why? How would this person encourage me to view the situation instead?
- If a friend had told me that they had faced (were facing or were about to face) the same situation as I faced and had made the same inference, what would I say to him/her about the validity of their inference and why? How would I encourage the person to view the situation instead?

Conclusion: *Based on what I know about my boss, the quality of my work that I submitted and what is going on in the company at this time, I think that it is highly unlikely that the reason why my boss wishes to see me is to criticize my work. The most likely explanation is that he wants to discuss aspects of my report in a non-critical way.*

Appendix 3

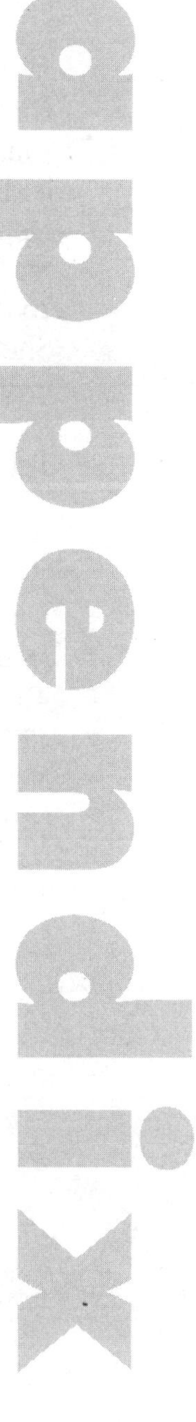

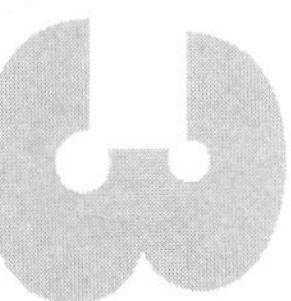

If you wish to consult an REBT therapist, here are some useful addresses and telephone numbers

United Kingdom
John Blackburn
AREBT
Department of Behavioural Psychotherapy
Sir Michael Carlisle Centre
75 Osborn Rd
Sheffield S11 9BF
England

Tel: +44 (0)114 2718699

Professor Windy Dryden
Tel: +44 (0)207 328 9687

United States of America
Albert Ellis Institute for REBT
45 East 65th Street
New York NY 10021
USA

Tel: +1 212 535 0822

Appendix 4

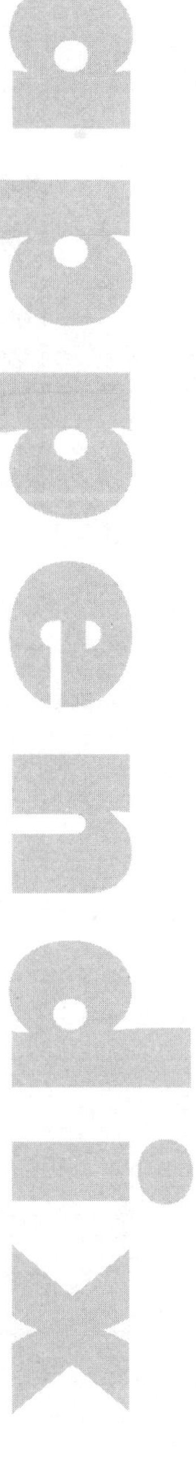

If you have specific emotional problems you might find it valuable to use some of the following books in conjunction with this workbook.

Dryden, W (1992) *The incredible sulk*. Sheldon: London (this book deals with the emotion of hurt as well as sulking).

Dryden, W (1994) *Overcoming guilt*. Sheldon: London.

Dryden, W (1996) *Overcoming anger: When anger helps and when it hurts*. Sheldon, London.

Dryden, W (1997) *Overcoming shame*, Sheldon: London.

Dryden, W (1998) *Overcoming jealousy*. Sheldon: London.

Dryden, W (2000) *Overcoming procrastination*, Sheldon: London.

Dryden, W (2000) *Overcoming anxiety*. Sheldon: London.

Dryden, W and Opie, S (2002) *Overcoming depression*. Sheldon: London.

References

Dryden, W (1994) *Ten steps to positive living*. Sheldon: London.

Dryden, W and Feltham, C (1995) *Counselling and psychotherapy: A consumer's guide*. Sheldon: London.

Rorer, LG (1999) Dealing with the intellectual-insight problem in cognitive and rational emotive behavior therapy. *Journal of Rational-Emotive and Cognitive-Behavior Therapy*, 17(4) 217–236.

Index